Medicines Missing Link

All about the fascinating subject of Metabolic Typing
and how the knowledge gained from it can be applied
for the improvement of health and well-being.

Medicine's Missing Link

Metabolic Typing and Your Personal Food Plan

Tom and Carole Valentine

THORSONS PUBLISHERS, INC.
Rochester, Vermont
—————— · ——————
Wellingborough, Northamptonshire

Thorsons Publishers, Inc.
One Park Street
Rochester, Vermont 05767

First U.S. edition 1987

Library of Congress Cataloging-in-Publication Data

Valentine, Tom.
    Medicine's missing link.

    Bibliography: p.
    Includes index.
    1. Metabolism. 2. Biochemical variation.
3. Health. I. Valentine, Carole. II. Title.
QP171.V35   1987   613.2   84-24063
ISBN 0-7225-1031-4

All quotations from the Kelley literature are reprinted with the kind
permission of Dr. William D. Kelley.

Printed and bound in Great Britain

10 9 8 7 6 5 4 3 2 1

Distributed to the book trade in the
United States by Harper and Row

Distributed to the book trade in Canada by Book Center, Inc.,
Montreal, Quebec

Distributed to the health food trade in Canada by Alive Books, Toronto
and Vancouver

Distributed to the book trade outside the United States and Canada
by Thorsons Publishing Group, Wellingborough, Northamptonshire,
England

Note to Reader

Contents

Chapter One:

One Man's Meat Is Another Man's Poison

The saying 'One man's meat is another man's poison,' coined by the Roman philosopher Lucretius, is more than two thousand years old, proving that people have long understood that no two human beings are exactly alike. Yet how quickly we have forgotten this ancient wisdom, especially when it comes to our diets and health.

Even the experts appear confused about this fact of life. For example, the late Nathan Pritikin and Dr Robert Atkins, noted American authorities on nutrition, both promoted a celebrated dietary regimen. Each was generally at the other's throat concerning the correctness of his own program and the incorrectness of the other's. What is the layman to believe? Which 'expert' is right?

As *Metabolic Typing* will illustrate, both experts were probably correct — *depending upon the metabolic types of the patients they surveyed for their reported results.* The fact is, you and I not only look different, we are different in more ways than we are alike. This book deals with the science of our differences.

At first glance, it would appear that learning about something as natural as 'what's good for us', would be easy to do. It isn't. Literally thousands of books have been written on the subject of health and nutrition, and so far, all it's done is raise more questions begging for answers. This book introduces some new thinking on an old theme as we probe into the research and application of knowledge about the different metabolic types.

There is controversy here, of course, as is usual in the arena of nutrition and health. But when all is said and done, this book may have supplied as many answers as it has aroused new questions.

Metabolic typing is a viable medical technology, and while it remains embryonic, the promise for the future is significant. The variables in human metabolism appear to be spread over a wide spectrum, so wide in fact, that, indeed, what is nourishing for one may be deleterious for another. This is one reason why so many fad diets prove to be more harmful than helpful in numerous cases.

Each of us has unique fingerprints, unique voiceprints, and a unique metabolism — our body's way of converting the food we eat into energy and cell growth. It's the old paradox — people are so much alike, and yet so curiously different. We certainly have no difficulty telling at a glance that a person is a person; obviously there are some general rules that encompass everyone. However, individuality is the hallmark of humankind, and each of us is totally unique. Just as it is impossible to dictate generalities in personal tastes, so is it impossible — and foolish — to dictate optimum human nutrition with blanket diet proposals, as our statistically-oriented society tries to do. Each person alone must be responsible for himself or herself. This means we must know ourselves — not only philosophically, but genetically and psycho-physiologically. Our biochemical inheritance from our parents, grandparents, and so forth, is uniquely our own.

Dr Roger J. Williams, one of the 'heroes' of this book and a pioneer in the study of biological individuality, describes in one of his books the experience that first aroused his keen interest in this field. Following a surgical operation he personally underwent many years ago, he writes, 'the doctor gave me a shot of morphine. It knocked out the pain, but I didn't go to sleep as the doctor intended me to do. Instead, my mind became so active that it was racing from one thought to the next. I was then given a larger dose of morphine. All night long, my mind raced faster and faster. I was suffering from continuous mental torture.'

Dr Williams' reaction to a basic drug differed from most other people's reaction. Although his doctor assured Williams that it was an 'idiosyncrasy', the fact of the biochemical difference intrigued the researcher's mind. However, he was not able to make sense of his individual reactions to established drugs until long after the experience.

Two decades after that 1930s episode, he read *The Atlas of*

Human Anatomy and noted that in illustrating the stomach, it did not present merely one picture of the stomach, but rather a number of drawings carefully made from autopsy specimens of 'normal' stomachs. In his book *The Wonderful World within You*, Dr Williams reproduced drawings of nineteen different stomachs (see Fig. 1.) and explained that stomachs differ not only in size and shape (just like ears and noses), but also in the structure and placement of the upper and lower valves, and that these valves may function differently (thereby treating food differently). Furthermore, Dr Williams learned, a Mayo Foundation study published sixteen years after his experience with morphine,

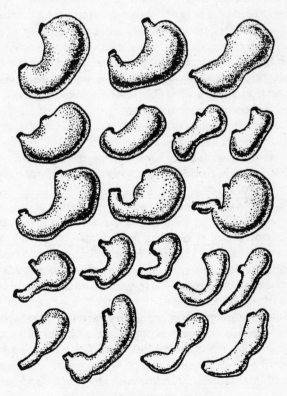

Figure 1. Nineteen stomachs
Reprinted with permission.

showed that stomachs differ widely in the composition of digestive juices. The juices actually differ more widely than the size and shapes of stomachs. Dr Williams wrote: 'In the case of the pepsin content of the gastric juice, the variation among normal adults is at least a *thousandfold*: although pepsin is of some importance as a digestive chemical, some people manage with very little of it. The hydrochloric acid content of normal gastric juices also varies widely' (emphasis added).

At about the same time that Dr Williams was making his observations of biological individuality, Dr George Watson of the University of Southern California completed studies that clearly indicated the existence of different types of metabolisms or 'energy exchanges within the body'. Dr Watson distinguished 'fast oxidizers' from 'slow oxidizers', and carefully monitored the effects on blood sugar levels and behavior. Slow oxidizers would generally become sluggish if they ate more food than they could metabolize. Fast oxidizers require slow-to-digest food in order to keep their blood sugar and hormone levels stable, thereby avoiding drastic mood changes. Much more on this later.

Such scientific studies are an important source of knowledge about metabolic differences. But no doubt many lay people have discovered these differences through personal experience. My wife, Carole, learned about them by observing the vast differences between her two sons.

Any parent who takes child rearing seriously can tell you that raising healthy kids is more than a full-time job; it's an around-the-clock operation. As a young mother more than two decades ago, Carole raised her sons, Sam and Jim, with old-fashioned European devotion. Her nurturing care gained momentum when her younger son, Jim, sustained chronic childhood ills and allergies to the point of missing major portions of the school year, and having the pediatrician prescribe tranquilizers. Furious that one so young should be prescribed powerful drugs, Carole discarded their sugary life-style and began a determined search for genuine health.

Sam and Jim are very much alike on the exterior. Both are tall, dark, and handsome. People who see them together often comment on the obvious fact they are brothers — perhaps even twins, although the notion of twins speaks of faulty observation.

However much they appear alike, the two brothers are nearly the full spectrum apart when it comes to metabolism.

'Jim! Don't eat that! You're going to make me sick!' Such exclamations were often blurted out by an astonished Carole when ten-year-old Jim snatched pieces of raw, red meat from the preparation table and ate them like a hungry savage. Jim has compulsively desired raw meat since his childhood, and today his body *requires* rare beef at least three times each week. The apparent requirement is more than a mere psychological craving. Jim's metabolic type turned out to be 'parasympathetic-dominant carnivore', when Carole finally placed herself and both boys on the Kelley Metabolic Ecology program in 1977-78.

Sam, on the other hand, gags at the thought of raw meat, and has a metabolism that does very well without even modest amounts of meat. He cannot do well on a purely vegetarian diet, but it wouldn't bother him if he never ate red muscle meats again.

The importance of these dietary variations within the same family struck Carole in the midst of her search for health when Sam was in high school and Jim in junior high. The family's food, their everyday nutrition, was stereotyped by the food industry, although the boys obviously had widely divergent nutritional requirements. She also became keenly aware that all those thousands of dollars spent on physicians had done absolutely nothing for Jim's health. As a result, Carole became a natural food 'nut'. Abandoning the concept of 'convenience' meals, she worked hard at preparing food for her family and eliminated all the 'junk' or refined, denatured foods available in supermarkets. She nurtured her boys from sickly adolescents to robust, ambitious, disciplined young men.

Carole's experience taught her what Roger Williams succinctly pointed out in his book *Biochemical Individuality*: that our modern, technically-oriented society is experiencing epidemic conditions of chronic and metabolic disease — disease that will eventually strike three out of every four of us. The highly refined and processed foods we consume are not only short of nutritional value, they afford little if any margin for the countless variables in individual metabolic needs.

Dr Williams' studies make a good case for his conviction that cancer, arthritis, heart disease, diabetes, alcoholism, and even schizophrenia are *all* based in 'cellular malnutrition'. Though he was not the first to champion research into individual differences, Dr Williams was surely the most prestigious scientist to do so. The discoverer of pantothenic acid and the first biochemist to be elected president of the American Chemical Society, Williams wrote: 'That malnutrition, unbalanced or inadequate nutrition, at the cellular level should be thought of as a major cause of human disease seems crystal clear to me. It is the inevitable conclusion to be drawn from the facts produced by decades of biochemical research.'

Dr Williams called for practical applications for identifying genetic individual differences and establishing some sort of 'metabolic profile' so that nutritional programs could be 'tailored to fit each individual's specific requirements'.

The man who actually established such a 'metabolic profile' is Dr William Donald Kelley, a dentist from Texas who is renowned today as a maverick cancer researcher. He saved his own life from deadly pancreas cancer more than twenty years ago, and during his personal struggle he learned more about health than he did disease.

Dr Kelley developed a system for determining at least ten distinct basic metabolic types. He is the founder of metabolic typing as a science and a new medical paradigm. One day our now sceptical establishment may well honor the work of this dedicated nutritional researcher.

Kelley didn't really invent anything new when he turned his concentration and energy to the subject of metabolic typing. He refined previous research, blended in a goodly amount of common sense, and founded a practical approach to individual differences. He developed the art of 'nonspecific metabolic therapy'. It is the *only* healing concept he will apply as a physician. Kelley explained his methods this way:

The technique is based upon the assumption that — if a person gives his or her body all the nutrients it needs, relieves its structural problems, stimulates the glands to do their jobs, cleans out any accumulated toxins and maintains the proper mental and emotional states — the body will be able to handle all sorts of problems, especially of a degenerative nature.

This method is, of course, the antithesis of conventional specialized medicine, which tries to isolate problems and treat them one at a time. Such accepted means of 'doctoring' are, I think, based upon a faulty premise: that the systems of the body function more or less independently, rather than in complete and continual dependence upon one another.

The human body is an amazingly adaptable organism. If all of a person's organs are working at anywhere near 100% efficiency, I believe the body chemistry is capable of rebalancing itself to eliminate almost any problem.

The only really effective way to treat an illness is to build health. The allopathic approach that is so common today is, at best, a temporary solution for degenerative problems.

Kelley's therapy modality, then, is knotted to his method for determining metabolic types, and that's what *Metabolic Typing* is all about.

Like most people who learn life's lessons well, Kelley learned about differing metabolic types from personal experience. After curbing his cancer with his own brand of vegetarian diet, supplements, and detoxification, he quite naturally felt enthusiastic about his success. His wife then developed serious health problems, so he immediately placed her on his strict vegetarian diet and supplementation program.

The great cure became a near total disaster! Suzi Kelley developed allergies, acute depression, and energy loss to the point of coma. She nearly died from Kelley's miraculous cure! Alarmed, he altered her diet and supplements to better suit her own particular metabolism, and she improved dramatically. 'That experience with Suzi', Dr Kelley has often testified, 'caused me to reformulate many of my ideas about nutrition.'

He then commenced a painstaking, methodical research into his patients as they related their unique preferences and feelings about diet, supplements, vitamins, and minerals. 'My eyes just hadn't been open to this obvious fact before', Kelley said. 'Some supplements and foods worked well for some people, while the same supplements and foods caused other people to feel terrible.'

Slowly he evolved classifications for people of different types, and eventually he devised a scale that numbered all the basic types. The extremes, he found, range from slow-oxidizing, sympathetic-dominant vegetarians at one end to fast-oxidizing, parasympathetic carnivores at the other. 'Sympathetic' and 'parasympathetic', you will learn later, refer to the autonomic nervous system — where, Kelley discovered, the *primary* reason for biochemical individuality lies.

In telling the tale of metabolic typing, this book does not dwell on the colorful controversy of Kelley's cancer research. However, Dr Kelley's name cannot be mentioned without cancer controversy creeping into the conversation. The reason for his notoriety is the story of actor Steve McQueen, a lung cancer victim who turned to Kelley when it was determined that malignant tumors had completely engulfed his right lung and spread to other areas of his chest and neck.

By 1980, Kelley had become known in alternative medicine circles as the world's leading authority on 'nontoxic' cancer treatment. When McQueen learned from his doctors that his cancer was 'hopeless', he visited Kelley's organic farm near Winthrop, Washington. Kelley made no predictions regarding a possible cure for the actor, but urged him to start total, around-the-clock therapy since every hour counted.

In an act of defiance suited to his public and private image, McQueen first staged a party before entering a Mexican facility dedicated to the Kelley program. When McQueen checked in on July 31, 1980, Dr Kelley regretted he had waited so long. 'He was in terrible shape', Kelley recalls. 'He had a blood clot in his arm and a tumor in his neck the size of an apple. He could hardly breathe, and he had no appetite.'

Despite the late stage and the long odds, McQueen agreed to co-operate and commenced treatment. He ingested massive doses of enzymes and vitamins to neutralize toxic agents in his body. He underwent a detoxification program of liver and gall-bladder 'flushes', kidney cleansing with diuretics and vegetable juices, and numerous coffee enemas, in which caffeine, passing through the portal vein directly into the liver, stimulates the liver's cleansing functions.

The medical establishment has attacked such programs derisively, and the therapy has been called 'Kelley's crazy laxative'. Kelley, however, accepted the research of Max Gerson, M.D., of New York, who showed that a tumor mass could be successfully treated by restoring the body's total metabolism. Gerson reasoned that coffee enemas stimulate bile secretions, which detoxify first the liver and then the rest of the body.

McQueen's treatments at Santa Maria, Baja California, came under attack. Helene Brown, a vocal opponent of what she regards as cancer quackery, said, 'This metabolic treatment is the craziest stuff you ever heard in your life . . . it's really a fraud.' Evidently she believed it would have been better for McQueen to do nothing after standard therapy practitioners called his case 'hopeless', and merely to die a miserable death.

McQueen started feeling better following six weeks of the rigorous therapy. He gained weight and strength and began taking short walks. The improvement was quite obvious even though McQueen was anything but an ideal, co-operative patient. He violated his diet often.

The media, especially the tabloids, sensationalized McQueen's treatment out of proportion. He wanted to live. He was a fighter. He told Mexican reporters: 'Mexico is showing the world this new way of fighting cancer through metabolic therapy . . . thank you for saving my life.'

Dozens of formerly 'terminal' cancer victims rallied on behalf of Kelley's therapy at a media event in Los Angeles on October 9, 1980. Reporters ignored the cured cancer patients' testimony to concentrate on McQueen.

On NBC-TV's *Today* show a doctor branded Kelley's therapy as 'rank quackery'. Kelley responded:

We have a good, scientific program, based on many years of research. Steve McQueen has upset the establishment by coming forward to challenge the chaotic medical care system in our country. Steve had been sent home to die. We have already extended his life by some two months beyond maximum predictions.

However, we are not at war with the medical community. We

are ready and willing to match our program on degenerative diseases against any other program endorsed by the National Cancer Institute, or the American Medical Association.

Kelley's supporters charged that McQueen's cancer grew unchecked in 1978-79 because antibiotics and drugs masked his serious condition.

McQueen felt so much improved after twelve weeks that he insisted upon driving back to his Santa Barbara, California, ranch. This rash decision dismayed Kelley and his staff. The establishment challenged Kelley's claim that McQueen was 'much improved', so Kelley allowed blind blood-test results (made on the blood of 'Don Schoonover', who was really Steve McQueen) to be made public. 'The first time this patient was tested', the laboratory report stated, 'he had three markers that were quite abnormal — very abnormal. But when I tested his blood the second time, some eight weeks later, all the markers were negative — that is to say, in the normal range. It was totally unbelievable for me to see such a tremendous clinical biochemical improvement.' The doctor signing that report was Emil Schandl, Ph.D., director of the CA Laboratory/Center in Dania, Florida. X-rays also confirmed that McQueen's tumors were indeed shrunken.

During his 'vacation' from the therapy, McQueen drank beer, smoked, and ate junk food, which demolished the benefits of much of the previous therapy. Complications developed, and it was determined that the tumor mass was putting pressure on the tubes running from McQueen's kidney to his bladder. Surgery was the only answer, despite the great risk.

Dr Cesar Santos Vargas, a Mexican heart and kidney specialist in Juarez, just across the Rio Grande from El Paso, Texas, was to do the surgery. McQueen, now more than eleven days off his metabolic regimen, was extremely weak.

Surgery removed tumors weighing more than three pounds, and most of the growths in McQueen's abdomen were no longer attached: they were dead masses easily lifted out. Following the surgery, McQueen was in good spirits and gave his well-wishers and physicians the 'thumbs up' sign. *'Lo hice!'* he cried in Spanish, meaning 'I did it!'

Fourteen hours later, on November 7, 1980, while sleeping under sedation, McQueen suffered a sudden heart seizure, followed by another that proved fatal. He died from a major risk factor in all surgery, an embolism, or blood clot, lodging in the heart.

The media, with help from establishment detractors of the Kelley program, distorted the truth. You've just read a recapitulation of the facts, and that's all the cancer controversy you'll receive from this book. Cancer, as we said earlier, taught Dr Kelley a lot about health.

Carole and I have watched the Kelley program grow, both separately and together, for nearly a decade. In 1974 I wrote about the Kelley cancer approach as a news journalist. In 1977 Carole placed herself and both her teenage sons on the Kelley nonspecific metabolic program. We trust that our experiences from the consumer's point of view will provide our readers with a balanced picture.

Since the credentialed experts are generally divided in their opinions on health and nutrition, how is it that uncredentialed authors stake a claim to writing a book that provides more answers than new questions? Carole and I are, admittedly, not institutionally credentialed — perhaps to our advantage. We are astute observers and skeptical reviewers, and we remain objective insofar as we have nothing to sell or promote save our books. We have no special-interest axes to grind; we're not on anyone's payroll, nor are we seeking government grants of any kind. We strive to be open, yet critical.

As learners and avid readers about health and nutrition, we learned early on that several factors contribute to confusion and controversy. One of the first problems is a lack of definition. What exactly is a 'healthy person'? To start out on the right foot, here's our definition:

The healthy person has energy in abundance and stamina for physical activity, including athletics, if he or she chooses.

The healthy person wakes up each morning feeling refreshed and moves about quickly after waking without stiffness or soreness.

The healthy person is a well-oiled machine with joints smooth, sinew taut, and bones sturdy; with hearty appetite, yet optimum weight for his or her skeletal structure.

The healthy person metabolizes food effectively and eliminates waste comfortably, with no need for chemical support such as laxatives.

The healthy person feels generally good and does not suffer undue highs or lows in levels of blood sugar.

The healthy person wards off infectious disease by virtue of a potent immune system, recovers rapidly when injured or sickened, and heals rapidly from bruises, contusions, and lacerations.

The healthy person has excellent vision, without corrective lenses, and excellent hearing.

The healthy adult person has perfect teeth and gums in a wide, strong jaw.

The healthy person has properly functioning glands and organs, which makes nature work overtime to degenerate his body with aging processes.

The healthy person, with a mate of equal health, produces children with vitality, strength, straight teeth, good eyesight, strong bones, firm constitutions, and psychological stability.

That's health! Have you ever met anyone who had it all? I haven't. Carole hasn't. It should be abundant, but perfect health is rare. We'd all like to be able to take it for granted, but once we stop kidding ourselves, we all know better. When health is absent or deficient, it's something we miss more than anything else.

To find people with optimum or near-optimum health, investigators have ranged all over the world. They've found some among isolated tribes and groups in obscure parts of the globe. The implications of these isolated findings may be an indictment of so-called civilized food processing.

Modern medical technology performs wonders but we're statistically clobbered by degenerative health conditions as our wonder medicine gives us longer life. The knowledge inherent in the study of basic metabolic types appears to be a missing link between wonder medicine and entrenched, though sophisticated, ignorance.

Another confusion factor sallies forth from the hodge-podge

of nutritional data generally available to the public. There are armies of experts in the field of nutrition, all waving a banner for their particular camp. One group, for example, argues against all animal fat. Many experts are staunch vegetarians, often for ethical or religious as well as health reasons. Some even claim that animal protein is toxic to humans. The opposite camp, however, argues that animal protein, especially egg, is the best source of protein available. One expert may stress that raw honey is no better or worse than refined sugar, while another argues that there is nothing wrong with refined sugar whatsoever. Many experts say that the benefits of vitamin supplements are grossly exaggerated by vitamin salespeople. Still others, with equally impressive credentials, retort that our foods are so refined and processed that they are 'denatured', depleted of necessary nutritional constituents, thus creating a need for supplementation.

Were you to read every available book on nutrition and health, you would end in utter confusion, unless you simply disregarded all the information distasteful to you. One of the important services rendered by the science of metabolic typing is that it separates one man's meat from the other man's poison by identifying individual differences.

Still another source for confusion stems from polarized propaganda put out by vested interests. On one side there is the food industry — giant corporations whose main concern is profit, not general health. These companies, generally speaking, have a powerful bureaucratic ally in various government agencies. This is a political fact of life attested to by the great number of corporate directors named to serve on government agencies, and the number of agency heads who move into high-level corporate positions.

Opposed to the corporate-government establishment stands a small army of lesser business interests striving to carve 'natural food' markets out of certain chinks in the corporate armor. These people also propagandize. They tell how bad all refined food products are, while projecting images of altruism and purity for themselves and their more 'natural' products — many of which are no less refined than giant corporation products.

The 'natural' versus 'denatured' argument spawns individuals with claims that they can 'cure' just about every disease, including cancer and multiple sclerosis, by feeding the victims certain herbs, grass juices, or other unorthodox remedies. Testimonials and claims from this tiny but vocal pressure group add to the confusion, making it seem as if these unusual treatments for specific disease conditions are 'good health practice' for normal, healthy people, too.

Herein lies one of the strengths of Dr Kelley's methodology. In determining his metabolic typing programs, Kelley noted the vast differences between a cancer victim and a relatively healthy person. He carefully segregated his research into the two distinct situations and eventually evolved his 'nonspecific' metabolic therapy. Kelley's idea is to let the body solve any specific problems that may be developing by providing optimum nutrition for that particular body metabolism.

In the case of advanced cancer, however, Kelley developed more 'specific' therapy in order to deal with the excess toxicity and other serious problems. By thus segregating his programs, Kelley accomplished much in overcoming inherent confusion, prejudice, and contradiction.

Finally, another source of reader confusion lies in the limited knowledge of the biological sciences. In another book in this series, *Applied Kinesiology,* we discuss how this muscle-testing modality has offered diagnostic insights unattainable within the limits of even modern, sophisticated medical know-how. No doubt science has made fantastic strides since the discovery of the double helix of DNA molecules, and we are entering the 'age of genetic engineering', perhaps even of 'cloning'; yet the causes of and controls for chronic metabolic disease continue to elude our understanding. Despite scientific advances, there remains a definite lack of hard knowledge concerning optimum human nutrition. Failing to account for the tremendous differences in human metabolism has been a major part of the problem.

Dr Melvin Page, who, like Dr Kelley, was a maverick dentist with a penchant for nutritional science, pointed out that society has only experienced about fifty years of serious inquiry into microbiology and metabolism, so it's fair to assume that fifty years from now we'll probably be laughing at many of our present-day assumptions. That's a key word — assumption. An assumption, although vital in research, is a 'made-up fact'. We must be aware that scientific assumptions, regardless of how impressively credentialed and professionally presented, are *not* general or eternal truths. For example, consider how widely accepted the theory of evolution is today, even though it is unproved and will likely always remain unproved. Today's 'science', utilizing the tenets of evolutionary theory, heaps assumption upon assumption to maintain workability. It is wise to recognize that.

In journalism, especially when delving into such controversial areas as health and nutrition, it pays to temper enthusiasm with a healthy skepticism. While I tend to want to believe, Carole always begins looking at new ideas with doubt. She has taught me that by beginning with doubt, one is likely to end with knowledge. Our faith in our fellow human beings is balanced by the knowledge that man is utterly fallible. That Dr Kelley, for example, is a diligent researcher who does his homework, is verified fact. That he has pioneered the greatest new wrinkle in the science of health and nutrition since the discovery of vitamins is still under consideration. The purpose of this book is to tell you what metabolic typing is all about and how you might apply this new learning to benefit yourself and your family.

Kelley didn't really find anything new. He merely looked at an old problem in a new, more open, and perhaps more determined way. Today most of the medical establishment would like to relegate Kelley to the quack heap. At the same time his supporters often want to canonize him. We are here neither to praise Kelley nor to bury him. We are here to relate the facts to the best of our ability.

Chapter Two:

Digestion — Metabolism's First Step

When Dr Kelley realized the tremendous difference between his metabolism and his wife's, he began diligently investigating the available research. Like all who strive to ferret out the facts from among diverse and controversial notions, Kelley encountered a lot of misinformation, partial truth, and distortion.

Although metabolism is the *sum total* of all the physical and chemical processes in the body, the digestion and assimilation of nutrition are obviously the major factor. We've all heard the shallow axiom that echoes from the halls of health food stores: 'You are what you eat.' Well, that turns out to be a partial truth. In reality you are what you metabolize — what your body assimilates and uses.

One school of thought encountered by nearly everyone who visits the hallowed bookshelves of the healthfood store is the notion of 'food combining'. The advocates of this approach to nutrition insist that the human digestive system is not capable of handling most of the combinations people enjoy eating. Meat and potatoes is considered a horrid mixture, for example. This school of nutrition quite seriously denies the built-in adaptability of our digestive and metabolic systems.

A large following developed around one particular group brandishing this thesis. The rationale stems primarily from a study made over a century ago. It seems that some poor fellow was shot in the stomach and his wound remained a gaping hole. His doctor evidently wanted to take advantage of this freak wound, so he paid the victim to allow him to study his digestion through the opening. This led to a 'classic' study of one man's digestive juices.

I can recall thinking all this information plausible years ago, until certain facts were called to my attention. First, even if the study were valid, it would have been accurate only for that man's particular system — and we have already seen how diverse human stomachs can be, not to mention the diversity of the gastric juice recipes involved in each. Second, the normal stomach reacts on a bolus of chewed and partially digested food that has traversed the esophagus. This particular study observed the stomach juice's action on foods dangled directly into the gaping hole on a string — quite a different matter. Third, even if the other objections weren't valid, the man being studied was obviously in a traumatized condition, so how could he demonstrate 'normal' stomach activity?

Kelley crossed the food-combining notions off his list of reliable sources of health information, for it is apparent from man's diverse nutritional history, around the world, that the digestive system is designed to cope with a wide spectrum of foods. Proper digestion handles all the combinations and variables.

Ah, but what is *proper* digestion? In truth, we must say that the modern digestive tract must be one of the wonders of the world. For several generations now, people in the so-called civilized world have brutalized their digestive tracts beyond nature's wildest dreams, doing things to themselves that ancient torture experts, seeking slow and devastating punishment, would surely have admired. Yet despite this brutality, modern people continue to bustle about busily (except when on sick leave); go on multiplying, albeit with more health problems than ever before; and apparently, in a large population statistical sense, are getting by 'normally'.

Dr Kelley and many other observers shudder at the thought of what the people of modern societies routinely do to their collective digestion. We agree. The constant health complaints of mainstream Americans, while they continue absorbing unmitigated junk, are infuriating to anyone who is knowledgable about nutritional health.

On the other hand, the medical establishment, propped up firmly by its massive insurance crutch, disdains any genuine critique of the glop we've stuffed into the mainstream trough. 'Eat a balanced diet', they say, 'of the four food groups' (taken directly from the supermarket shelves in their denatured, additivized, refined form) 'and you'll do nicely'.

Dr Kelley's method for establishing metabolic types would have been far easier to accomplish had he limited his research to various ethnic and tribal groups found in isolated pockets around the world. He would have encountered people in excellent health, with vigor and longevity. Of course, they would have been isolated from the refinements of sophisticated, technically enriched foods.

It certainly wasn't easy for Kelley to extrapolate the distinctions between metabolic types while dealing primarily with Americans exhibiting complaints of degenerative disease.

When Dr Kelley began to classify people into the various metabolic types, he realized that the key to discovery lay in the dominance of one or the other of the two branches of our autonomic nervous systems. In the next chapter we'll delve into the details of the anabolic-catabolic, or sympathetic-parasympathetic, dominance roles, but at this point a clear picture of our collective digestive processes, and the West's love affair with indigestion, may lead to a better understanding of health and nonhealth in the light of the thesis being presented.

The first step in everyone's digestive process is *chewing* — the step the 'classic' food-combining study overlooked. Incidentally, all you need do is look around a restaurant and you can see that this initial exercise alone is rife with individual differences.

People seem to have forgotten the importance of chewing. Seldom does one overhear parents reprimand their children for failing to chew their food properly. Actually, my parents did not admonish me to do so nearly as severely as my grandparents did: (If anyone is prompted to ask, 'What do "old folks" know, anyway?', let him recall the fact that they lived to *be* 'old folks'.)

In this era of the rebirth of preventive medicine and holistic health, it is depressing to see hordes of people frequenting fast-food services of all kinds in order to gulp down standardized, refined, additivized, denatured products sold as food. It is even sadder to see young people dashing from an 'aerobics' class to a fast-food outlet for some hasty gulping and guzzling, followed by a cigarette.

The majority of people today simply cannot eat food without swilling down some sugary beverage. This, of course, is a direct assault on the digestive system, regardless of metabolic type. In fact, this collective habit is indulged *irrespective* of metabolic type, which is something few people have yet heard of, and fewer still seem to accept. Dr Kelley has proved that indiscriminate consumption leads to miserable health conditions in many people.

But, you may say, 'everybody does it', so it can't be all bad. Besides, most people do get a little something from all four food groups at some time or other during the week, don't they? Just what the doctor ordered!

Can it be that our young people are being allowed to sacrifice their health in order to bolster the economy? Think about that! Without regard for individual differences, millions upon millions of people in the world today — and not just teenagers — do not eat food without washing it down with various beverages, mostly soft drinks. This habit is a commercial bonanza, in more ways than one. Not only does it help make the soft-drink industries the darlings of Wall Street, it adds billions to the coffers of the manufacturers of digestive aids.

First, look at the economics of the sugary swill — so cheap to make — that modern people guzzle. It started in about 1849 when 1.1 persons across America managed to drink a twelve-ounce container of soda pop in one year's time. By 1909 the industry noted that the per-capita consumption of pop was 10.8 bottles per year. By 1978 that per-capita figure had risen to 382.7 bottles of pop — that's more than one a day for every man, woman, and child in the United States, and a lot of us never touch the stuff! For a more vivid proof of this statistic, one has only to look at the numbers and sizes of bottles of soda pop meandering through supermarket checkout lines.

Incidentally, you may have noticed the big switch of emphasis in television commercials to the 'no-caffeine' formula. The marketplace is slowly catching on to the notion of toxicity, at least in one category.

Swilling has replaced chewing in the land of the free, who are going to need to be brave to endure the health degeneration they shall surely reap. And, even though the idea of food-combining taboos doesn't apply when we are dealing with natural foods and adaptable metabolisms and proper digestion coupled with good habits, the combination of highly refined carbohydrates (white flour, white sugar, white rice) and concentrated proteins (meat, eggs, cheese) will certainly tax a brutalized modern digestive tract.

One would think that Americans would get smart, en masse. The evidence is everywhere that a serious problem exists. For example, the second half of the economic picture that our careless eating habits create is the amount of money generated by the 'health care industry'. As a nation, the United States generates more money through health care than it does through all but two production categories. Agribusiness is still number one; manufacturing is still number two; but 'health care' is a fast-closing third. Americans spend better than 10 per cent of their *gross national product*, or roughly $600 million *per day,* on 'health care'.

And, if such cost figures aren't enough to wake people up, how about the hidden message of those television commercials that target problems with digestion? Reason, if you will, this way: prime-time commercial costs are staggering, implying that products that are advertised, over and over again, during that prime time, must, therefore, be exceptionally profitable — which means people buy lots of them. And we generally buy what we think we need. America, obviously, needs digestion help.

We'll not bore you with further statistics. Suffice it to say that Americans spent nearly $40 *billion* on over-the-counter and prescription 'remedies' in 1984, and the pharmaceutical industry never looked healthier. The marketing folks down at the friendly drug factory know that digestive abuse accounts for 18 per cent of that huge market. That means Americans purchase about $8 billion worth of antacids, laxatives, and cathartics each year.

What does it all mean? Dr Kelley tosses out several interesting statistics — not generally known, nor highly publicized. Now, we certainly don't want to throw statistics around as a bureaucrat would. I'm always reminded of the statistician who drowned in a river with an average depth of one foot. Statistics are such curious critters that a person may earn a doctorate, perhaps even a Nobel Prize, for merely coming up with a truly viable way to 'analyze' them. Regardless, let's share some general statistics that Kelley has assembled in his literature to paint a 'frightening picture of our current health status'.

- 999 out of 1,000 people today are malnourished.
- Birth defects in the U.S. have tripled since 1956.
- About 80 per cent of America's population suffers from degenerative diseases.

- The National Cancer Institute of America has found that 'diet and nutrition appear to account for the largest number of human cancers'.
- Only a few years ago, accidents were the major cause of death in children under the age of fifteen, but today the number-one cause is cancer.
- One person dies of cancer every eighty seconds in the United States.
- Degenerative disease conditions, such as cancer, diabetes, heart disease, hypoglycemia, eczema, emphysema, arthritis, and ulcers occur in more and more *children* each year.
- Chronic illness is responsible for more than 80 per cent of the total cases of disability in the U.S.
- Each year the United States drops lower on the list of 'health of nations'.

Dr Kelley dedicated his life to the pursuit of genuine health and preventive medicine, and his contribution of 'metabolic ecology' may well be the key to ultimately reversing the slipping and sliding health statistics.

Many of the 'new age' health programs now being sold to a small aware segment of society are doomed to failure because the metabolic differences, and the effects of these differences on our digestion of available foods, are not yet understood or recognized by many.

Digestion means the process of changing nutritious food into needed products to be absorbed into the blood and assimilated upon delivery to all the cells of the body. Not only are most Americans and other modern peoples in the world (look how the Chinese delighted in getting Coca-Cola and other franchise operations) unaware of the importance of digestion, they are ignorant of the vital differences in individual metabolism. This can be a deadly, degenerating combination of ignorance.

While in the process of writing this book, I met an anesthesiologist and mentioned the subject I was working on. 'I can't relate to that at all', he responded when I sketched metabolic typing. That medical doctor may be forgiven for his education, and the rest of us may be forgiven for our previous ignorance and sometimes stupidity. Most of my life I felt confident that I possessed what we used to call in my macho youth a 'strong stomach'. I'm glad I met Carole and learned some sensible healthy thinking at about age forty-four. You see, my 'strong stomach' had turned on me. Carole taught me, as she had taught herself and her sons, what she had learned from a well-known health personality, Dale Alexander. While millions of Americans spell relief 'antacid', as TV commercials suggest, Alexander spells relief 'eating without drinking'.

No matter which metabolic type you turn out to have, your digestion·and metabolism faculties will operate better without dilution. For years and years, Alexander, the advocate of cod liver oil (earning him the sobriquet 'The Codfather'), has harangued his audiences on the deadly sin of drinking water — especially iced water — or other liquids while chewing and eating.

Carole has insisted upon following Alexander's dictates, and it has apparently paid dividends. Our family does not drink with the meal, and we wait a full hour following a light meal before drinking anything, or two full hours following a heavy meal. It is an excellent digestive practice (cured a number of my former gastric problems far better than antacids ever did) and also an outstanding *disciplinary* practice — not too harsh, not too easy.

Now, if nutritional ignorance is so widespread and if the typical diet is so junk-food-ridden, then why do some individuals not only survive to age ninety-eight, but have to be killed falling off a horse coming home from a brothel? We've all heard that yarn. In my own family tree there was an Uncle Tom, who was terribly obese, smoked roll-your-own cigarettes at an industrial clip, devoured the fattiest pork and bacon dishes several times a week, and never ate one of those fatty meals without several cups of coffee washing it down. The Grim Reaper finally called on old Tom some time in his nineties, while he was out sawing logs.

Those kinds of stories, which are rare enough to be excellent conversation pieces, tell us several things, but certainly not that there is nothing wrong with modern dietary practices. Yes, we must admit that even today there are some genetic constitutions that appear to defy the odds. These individuals seem to cope with denatured, refined, additivized, swillwashed food product and never be the worse for wear. Well, if true, the old yarn tells us that there certainly must be different metabolic types.

Besides, Uncle Tom's children didn't necessarily do as well when it came to health. Of course, Tom probably had the benefit of thirty years or so of unrefined, more natural foods since he managed to live in less pre-packaged times.

My own grandparents all lived to an old age, especially my maternal 'grandmother', who lasted until her ninety-fourth year. My father, however, succumbed to cancer of the colon in his late sixties. His brothers both died before him, and it may be said that despite rugged, hard-working lives, robust health was not necessarily a hallmark of that generation when compared with their parents.

The statistics on degeneracy speak of a sad state of affairs for the very young. It worsens with each generation. How can unhealthy parents reproduce healthy children? And we should not be fooled by talk that our youthful athletes are bigger, stronger, and faster than ever. These are statistical distortions. Not only has the population base from which athletes are spawned increased considerably, providing increasingly more bodies to choose from for athletics, but drugs and chemical stimulants and some aspects of nutritional science seem to play a key role of their own in the 'bigger and better' syndrome.

Watch closely; even the healthy-looking young person today requires a candy bar or some form of stimulant to maintain 'normal' energy levels. Carole and I are not impressed with the empty claims of 'bigger and better' youth. We take the opposite view from the vast majority.

Evolution theory, applied to adaptive mankind, demands a constant though barely perceptible change for the better — the 'clod to God' thesis. This theory, though full of holes, is accepted in modern biological science circles. However, the evidence, as we see it, indicates *devolution* and degeneration, which is more in line with the physical law of entropy — that law which states that everything in the material universe is coming apart, not improving.

Several years ago, I uttered an unthinking opinion to an audience at a health gathering. I told them that evolution would eventually produce a breed of humans capable of thriving on junk food. I believed in evolutionary theory religiously then. Imagine, if you will, a future athlete performing fantastic feats while nourished only on twenty-first century soda pop, microwaved pizza, and synthetic chocolate.

Of course that cannot happen, despite the beliefs of many. In order for that prediction of mine to be valid, the human body would have to change too drastically to survive. The amino acids, fatty acids, minerals, vitamins, and other nutrients required to build body cells would have to be evolved into totally different compounds. The chances against such a change occurring are astronomical.

No doubt our bodies have a remarkable *adaptability,* but this should not be mistaken for evolution. Our species experiences all kinds of genetic alteration and blending to cope with the varied environmental encounters, but not to the extremes required by evolutionary adherents.

What legacy, then, might we be leaving future generations? Dr Francis Pottenger, now of the Price-Pottenger Nutrition Foundation in San Diego, completed several long-term animal studies — primarily his famed 'cat studies' — during the 1940s and 1950s. His studies showed that animals on totally refined and processed foods deteriorated to the point of failure to reproduce within a span of only a few generations. To us, if the present-day policies of 'economics before health' and 'convenience before care' continue unabated, our world may not need a nuclear holocaust to leave an international population of retarded mutants.

If preventive medicine is going to have any beneficial, long-range effect, it had better pick up a head of steam among society soon.

Dr Kelley's research and resultant Metabolic Ecology program provide a significant, far-reaching perspective from which to begin improving general health. Let's consider this thesis, before it's too late.

Chapter Three:

The Autonomic Nervous System — Key to Your Individual Needs

Since metabolism is the sum total of all your body's processes for using raw materials — air, light, water and food — to form chemical energy, the practice of metabolic typing is not absolute. It's not a hard science like arithmetic, but it's not squishy like psychology or sociology, either. Dr Kelley's classifications and metabolic types are based on careful evaluations of physiological processes made over many years.

Your body is a self-regulating system which is truly one of the wonders of nature. The mechanism for this self-regulation is the nervous system. People have a lot of nerve, and it's a good thing. The key to your unique individual metabolism lies in the operations under the control of that part known as the autonomic nervous system.

Sometimes people may say 'automatic nervous system', and in a sense that's almost the same thing as 'autonomic', except that 'automatic' is for supermarket doors and 'autonomic' is for describing the system of nerves, proprioceptors, and ganglia that controls all the goings-on in our glands, organs, and smooth muscle. The system operates on its own — thus autonomic or autonomously. We do not need to consciously think about our autonomic operations at all. Probably we would botch them up in a few seconds if we could think about them.

The important role in our health played by the autonomic nervous system is recognized by the ancient arts known as yoga and acupuncture. Neither of these two practices would bear any weight if the autonomic nervous system did not directly and thoroughly oversee and operate our metabolic functions.

Acupuncture meridians appear to be patterns of vital energy

flowing and ebbing around our bodies much like the invisible electrical fields outside high-tension wires. Acupuncturists have learned the relationships of these meridians to physiology, especially the autonomic nervous system, and are therefore able to perform various feats of anesthesia and healing.

Yoga has been practiced in various forms under different names around the world, but it is associated primarily with Hinduism and is a spiritual as well as a physical and mental discipline. The yogi practices various physical postures, concentrates on control of the breath (autonomic function), and eventually obtains a measure of control over parts of the autonomic nervous system's functions. A practiced yogi with years of experience may actually alter certain body functions, including heartbeat and circulation.

Whether this 'conscious control' is superior to autonomic function is a matter that we won't argue here. We merely wish to point out that the autonomic nervous system is indeed the key to health and to individual metabolic types. Researchers have concentrated on autonomic nervous systems — not their own, other people's — and learned that *each individual's system functions uniquely according to the size and number of cells in his or her organs and glands.*

Some of the difference is obvious. For example, many people appear to build up energy reserves at a greater rate than others. Then there are those who seem to deplete or use up their energy as fast as it comes in. In some psychogenic illnesses, like anorexia, owing to emotional stresses the system may deplete energy even faster than raw material comes in. Most of us, however, appear balanced — we keep some and spend some.

Carole is a lithesome, slender woman, yet she eats about as much as I do of the same kinds of nutrition. Her body uses it all up nicely in a balanced way on a minimum of exercise. My body, by contrast, enjoys the food so much that it keeps it around, and around, and around. I'm forced to exercise vigorously just to keep some of the excess away.

Dr Kelley reviewed the existing research on metabolism and individual uniqueness, then conducted intensive, long-term research of his own in order to develop a system for accurately classifying the various patterns into basic metabolic types. After thoroughly analyzing the physiological, psychological, and behavioral aspects of thousands of individuals, Kelley designed effective nutritional support programs suited to the needs of each of the basic types.

The Kelley metabolic typing system first divides everyone into one of three general categories based entirely upon the autonomic nervous system in general. People, Kelley learned, may be *sympathetic*-dominant, *parasympathetic*-dominant, or balanced between the two.

The sympathetic and parasympathetic systems are two distinct functional modes of the autonomic nervous system. Sometimes the terms *anabolic* and *catabolic* are used to describe the particular mode of metabolic function being discussed. Parasympathetic anabolism and sympathetic catabolism are, if you will, merely professional jargon for put-ins and take-outs.

The sympathetic-catabolic system marshals the forces of your body energy. It takes what it needs and uses it. When the old adrenaline starts to flow and you are excited, tensed for flight or fight, as they say, your sympathetic system is in high gear.

The parasympathetic-anabolic system is responsible for building up, or 'putting in', the needs of your body — processing raw materials into cells, for example. The parasympathetic system is associated with rest and repair and with our vitally important immune system.

The human being is an incredible creature to contemplate and certainly deserves the title 'highest order of life', which we've bestowed on ourselves. A junior high school teacher of mine once told our class that 'a good engineer could design a more efficient human body, but we'll have to make do with what nature gave us'. I cannot fathom the gall of such a statement today. The truth is, engineering at its best can't come up with an automatic supermarket door that will last more than a few years.

Figure 4, a diagram of Kelley's 'metabolic types' clearly shows the relationship of all ten basic types to each other. Horizontally we see the tendencies toward dominance by one side of the autonomic system or the other. Vertically the chart indicates the body's tendencies toward efficiency or inefficiency in metabolizing raw materials.

Ideally, in Kelley's system, each person should be a ten, having a perfectly balanced, highly efficient metabolism. But few people

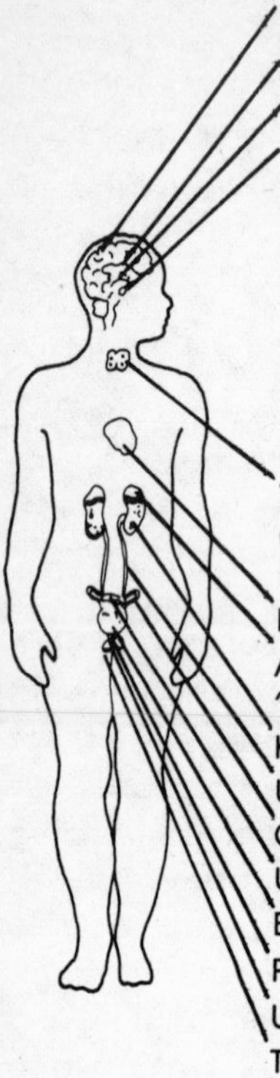

LEFT BRAIN: verbal and analytical capacity

Posterior Lateral HYPOTHALAMUS

THALAMUS: switchboard to higher brain centers

ANTERIOR PITUITARY GLAND works in balance with thyroid, adrenal, and gonads; produces the following hormones.
1. GH (growth hormone): bone and general body growth, physical shape
2. TSH (thyroid stimulating hormone): stimulates formation and growth of thyroid gland
3. ACTH (adrenal cortex stimulating hormone): stimulates formation of adrenal cortex hormones
4. LH, FSH, beta-LPH

THYROID produces thyroxin, increases activity of cells, regulates metabolism and calcitonin for depositing calcium in bones and tissues

HEART

ADRENAL MEDULLA (inner) produces adrenaline, controls 'fight or flight' reaction

KIDNEYS

URETER

OVARIES ♀

UTERUS

BLADDER ♂

PROSTATE

URETHRA

TESTES

GENITO-URINARY SYSTEM: Kidneys
Bladder
Urethra
Ureters

REPRODUCTIVE SYSTEM: Ovaries
Uterus
Testes
Prostate

Skeletal system
Muscle system
Cardiovascular system
Neuromuscular system
Urinary system
Reproductive system
Ligaments, connective tissue
Arteries
Veins
Capillaries
Calcium metabolism

Figure 2. Physical aspects dominated by the sympathetic nervous system.

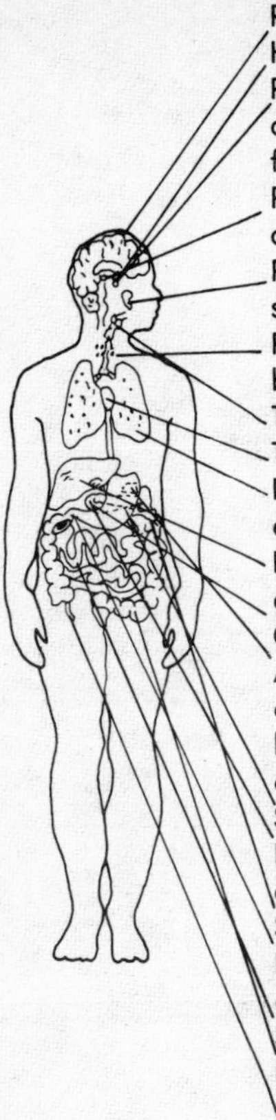

RIGHT BRAIN: intuitive and spatial capacities
HYPOTHALAMUS: anterior medial
POSTERIOR PITUITARY GLAND produces two hormones, controls water metabolism, blood pressure, kidney function, smooth muscle action.
PINEAL GLAND is responsive to light, reproductive cycles and pigmentation.
PAROTID GLAND helps conserve DNA material, stimulates parasympathetic organs and glands.
PARATHYROIDS: Parathormone releases calcium from bones.
TONSILS: immune system organ, infection warning system
THYMUS: immune system organ
LUNGS: carbon dioxide, oxygen and waste gases exchange from blood
LIVER: energy storage, food processing, detoxification, etc.
GALLBLADDER: bile storage
ADRENAL CORTEX (outer) produces several hormones; controls swelling, inflammation, sodium potassium balance; glucocorticoids stimulate production of carbohydrates from proteins, etc.
STOMACH produces hydrochloric acid for digestion
PANCREAS: stimulated by vagus nerve; produces digestive enzymes; aids carbohydrate metabolism
SPLEEN: immune system organ, blood regulation
DUODENUM: first part of small intestine; contains openings of pancreatic duct and common bile duct
SMALL INTESTINE: digestion and absorption
LARGE INTESTINE: B vitamins manufactured, water absorbed
APPENDIX: immune system organ, regulates blood cell production

Bone marrow (regulates blood cell production)
Digestive system
Immune system (defends against environmental stress and toxins)
Lymphatic system (stores poisons, extra nutrients)
Respiratory system
Excretory system (skin, lungs, lymph, colon, liver, kidney, bladder)
Carbohydrate metabolism
Cholesterol metabolism
Fat metabolism
Protein metabolism
Starch metabolism

Figure 3. Physical aspects dominated by the parasympathetic nervous system.

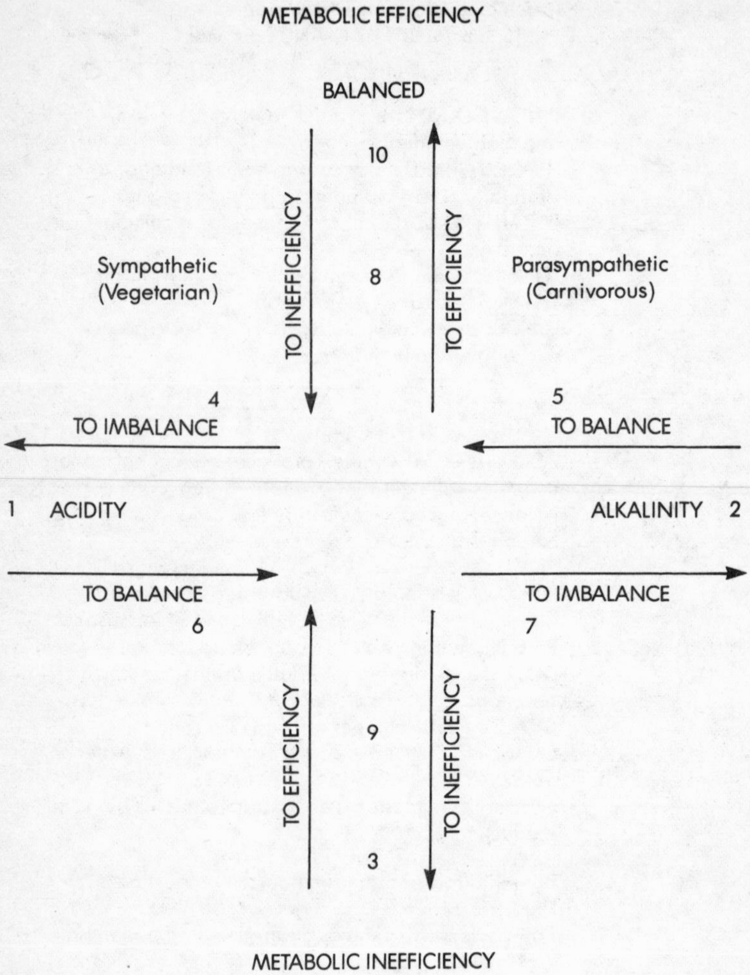

METABOLIC EFFICIENCY

BALANCED

10

8

Sympathetic
(Vegetarian)

TO INEFFICIENCY

TO EFFICIENCY

Parasympathetic
(Carnivorous)

4
TO IMBALANCE

5
TO BALANCE

1   ACIDITY

ALKALINITY   2

TO BALANCE
6

TO IMBALANCE
7

TO EFFICIENCY

TO INEFFICIENCY

9

3

METABOLIC INEFFICIENCY

Figure 4. Metabolic types. Reprinted from the Kelley Book, with permission.

would actually be typed as 'a perfect 10'. This type, according to Kelley, is

> a person who can eat a wide variety of foods and take a wide variety of supplements, but does not require a large amount of anything. Type 10's are the people with super-efficient metabolisms. Their bodies are so incredibly efficient that they need very small amounts of food. If they eat a normal meal, they feel more than satisfied. They can eat half as much as any other metabolic type, and be fully satisfied and unbelievably energetic. They do well on *any* food, but often prefer raw fruits, vegetables, whole grains and cheese.

In December of 1983, after years of checking and double-checking his research, Dr Kelley added types 11 and 12 to the ten basic metabolic types. Like type 10 metabolizers, types 11 and 12 have exceptionally efficient metabolisms. However, they will never be perfectly balanced or be able to eat all the foods that type 10 people do. Genetically, type 11 is sympathetic-dominant and type 12 is parasympathetic-dominant, and they will always remain so.

Although the Kelley Metabolic Ecology program strives to bring individuals toward balance, Kelley's research has convinced him of the fact that there are, indeed, some genetically determined dominance factors that cannot change.

Looking at Figure 4, you can quickly spot the positions of the ten basic types in relation to balance and efficiency indicated by the two sliding scales (arrows), one moving vertically the other horizontally.

Vertically we can see that type 8 is in the center (balanced) and tends to be efficient, but not superefficient. This is the type assigned to the greatest number of people today. Type 8 metabolizers, Kelley explained, have

> fairly healthy bodies; bodies that can adapt to a wide variety of stresses, and yet remain stable. These individuals have autonomic nervous systems with a wide range of adaptability, and they may need a wide variety of foods each day. This permits them to attempt to obtain a large variety of nutrients, required

to operate their bodies efficiently. Nutritional supplements for type 8 metabolizers, like their food, must cover a wide spectrum.

In the 'balanced but inefficient' category we see numbers 9 and 3. This means that while type 9 and type 3 metabolizers have the two branches of their autonomic system working together in a normal balance of glandular or organ activity, their efficiency is gradiently worsening.

Type 3 metabolizers, Kelley stressed, are balanced:

that is, their sympathetic and parasympathetic nervous systems are functioning in balance equally well, but they come with bodies that are very inefficient. No matter what foods or supplements they take in, they are generally going to use only about 10% to 15% of the nutrition. These type 3's find it difficult for their individual cells to obtain adequate nutrition. All refined, processed, synthetic foods and food additives must be avoided at all times. Type 3 metabolizers of necessity must take larger quantities of nutritional supplementation to maintain their nutritional health than any other type. They must eat food prepared in such a manner as to be easily digested. They should have a wide variety of food, which enables them to get the wide spectrum of nutrients their bodies require.

Unfortunately, due to the stress of modern living and agribusiness, more and more Americans who have inherited good bodies have so exhausted and destroyed their bodies that they are now functioning in the type 3, 6 or 7 range. It would take a supreme effort to rebuild and repair these bodies and put them back into good health again.

That's quite a thumbnail sketch of a metabolic type. Let's think about that for a moment.

Imagine, if you will, a type 3 metabolizer putting himself on the Nathan Pritikin program. The Pritikin program targets cholesterol, so dairy products, eggs, butter, red meats, and even moderate amounts of lean fish or fowl are unacceptable. The type 3, who feels bad anyway, is going to assimilate only portions of the skimpy, fat-free, anticholesterol diet, and his need for supplementation is going to remain unchanged. However, Pritikin emphasized that 'a natural diet has more vitamins than you can use. The public is tremendously oversold on vitamins; only about one person in a million needs vitamins. But, taking care of your heart, ah, that's something different.'

First, I'm compelled to ask, where did Pritikin get the statistic that only one person in a million needs vitamins? Second, although Carole and I generally agree that vitamin commercialism is often beyond the realm of good sense, we also realize there is a definite need for nutritional supplementation in modern society because of the denatured quality of our primary food source — the depleted, chemicalized farming soils — and also because *many* individuals have poor metabolisms and do not assimilate nutrients well. Therefore, supplementation is vital.

Clearly, certain individual metabolisms simply cannot be assumed to fit into a generalized category, such as the Pritikin program. Additionally, today's refined, processed supermarket foods may be convenient and sanitary, but they do pose definite problems for large numbers of the population — and, we argue, the health statistics support that indictment.

Because Kelley's type 8 metabolizers account for the greatest number of people he has evaluated — indicating that the broadest category indeed fits the slot most of us would label 'normal' — we may assume things are as they should be and the Kelley metabolic typing system stands up to logic.

The final type in the balanced category, type 9 metabolizers, Kelley indicates are the 'most difficult to understand.' He explains:

If these people had a choice, they would always prefer cooked food. Working with these individuals through the years has led me to the conclusion that they truly cannot do well on raw foods. Evidently they have mutated somehow to the point that they need cooked food to be satisfied. They generally require 70% cooked food and may comfortably handle no more than 30% raw food. Type 9 metabolizers do best when they can have a smorgasbord three or four times a week. In other words, if they eat a little of everything, they function better.

I can sense the stirrings of curiosity as the pages turn and readers wonder, 'What type am I?' The problem with going through thumbnail sketches of the various metabolic types is that each time we read one we begin to think, 'Aha, that's like me!' For example, the cooked-food part of type 9 seemed to strike a strong chord here. Raw foods have very little appeal to me, although I do enjoy green salads.

I remind you that at the beginning of this chapter we pointed out that metabolic typing was more analytical than precise like arithmetic. In metabolic typing we encounter the dynamics of constant change, which everybody faces every day, and the variables outweigh the absolutes. Kelley's actual typing-by-computer programs prints out for each individual the percentages that his or her particular metabolism appears to reflect each of the basic types. More of this later; first let's tackle the horizontal sliding scale of the metabolic type chart — the vegetarian to meat-eater scale.

Chapter Four:

The Ten Metabolic Types

For years and years, it seems, the debate between advocates of vegetarianism and hearty beef eaters has followed me around, and for years and years, I didn't have enough perspective to deal with the controversy intelligently, so I resorted to the response 'to each his own!'

It turns out that my liberal compromise was an intelligent one in light of the differences in human metabolic types.

Vegetarians, in our experience, tend to scold meat eaters for their carnivorous tastes and to dismiss the notion that meat has any virtue as a 'health' food. Most healthfood stores tend to favor vegetarianism, although most seem to cater to 'ovo-lacto vegetarians', who eat eggs and milk products, which of course are animal foods.

Carole and I have often resented the 'mystic vegetarian' approach that accosted us as we shopped at a local healthfood store. We prefer natural to denatured, organic to chemicalized, pure to additivized foods, so we like to shop where such products (including certain meats) are available. To do so comfortably, we have often had to bite our tongues when confronted with the beliefs of certain staunch vegetarians. These vegetarians tend to be more emotional than logical, which would be fine if only they acknowledged it and didn't insist on the unimpeachable rationality of their beliefs. Generally, however, that is not the case. Eating meat means killing animals, and that is the basis of most of the antimeat propaganda heard in the healthfood stores. Fortunately, Kelley's metabolic typing lifts the issue of meat eating out of the morass of emotion and sentimentality and allows us to consider it dispassionately.

On the metabolic type chart (Figure 4) in Chapter 3, the

parasympathetic-dominant (carnivorous) types are to the right. The sliding scale is horizontal, and the extremes are represented by types 1 and 2. The type 1 person is running off the chart to the left, away from balance. This person is a highly sympathetic-dominant individual. Note that according to the chart this person tends toward acidity rather than a balance between the acid and alkaline factors.

The opposite is type 2, running off the scale to the right, toward alkalinity. The acid-alkaline balance in our bodies is very important. With certain functional exceptions, our body systems should be like water in a swimming pool, neither acid nor alkaline. In terms of health in today's society, these two extremes are neither good nor bad — they are simply extreme. However, Kelley's Metabolic Ecology program always strives to bring individuals back toward the center, to balance. A person's particular type is defined only after considering a wide range of physiological and metabolic functions, which may be said to differ in efficiency, expression, and importance from type to type. Once an individual type is accurately determined, the proper foods, vitamins, minerals, and other supplements, such as enzymes and glandular extracts, may be prescribed. Equally important, the supplements and foods to be *avoided* may be pointed out.

Sympathetic-Dominant Metabolizers: Types 1, 4, and 6

The sympathetic-dominant metabolizers, types 1, 4, and 6, tend to have good muscle tone and well-developed musculature. Their hearts may beat, normally, a little fast. Constipation is an ever-present plague. Frequently they suffer from insomnia, hypertension, and hyperactivity. They are often *driven* emotionally. These people are *prone* to the following conditions:

Achlorhydria   Diminished appetite
Acidosis   Arteriosclerosis
Acne   Arthritis (rheumatoid)
Alcoholism   Bleeding (slow clotting)
Anemia   High blood pressure
Angina pectoris   Infrequency of bowel
Anxiety   movements

Boils
Bone pain
Rapid breathing
Buergers disease
Bursitis
Cancer
Canker sores
Slow metabolism of
   carbohydrates
Caries (cavities)
Cataracts
Chorea
Tight circulation
Ulcerative colitis
Conjunctivitis
Constipation
Cystitis
Dehydration
Diabetes
Slow digestion
Dizziness
Earache
Easily upset emotionally
Lack of endurance
Low energy reserve
Epilepsy
Cool extremities
Dry eyes
Slow fat metabolism
Food feels heavy in stomach
Function well in hot weather
Febrile diseases
Gag easily
Sweet-smelling gas
Glossitis
Goiter
Gout
Halitosis

Heart attacks
Heartburn
Heart arrhythmia
Headaches (migraine,
   tension)
Rapid healing of bones
Slow healing of tissues
Hemorrhoids
High temperatures
Hyperirritability
Hypertension
Hyperchlorhydria
Indigestion
Bacterial infections
Insomnia
Ketosis
Kidney infections
Kidney stones
Night restlessness in legs
Dry mouth
Myocarditis
Nephritis
Nervous strain
Numbness
Poor oxygen metabolism
Unusual sensitivity to pain
Pellagra
Peyronie's disease
Photophobia
Pneumonia
Poor protein metabolism
Fast pulse
Purpura
Rheumatic fever
Sensitivity to light
Sensitivity to shots
Dry, thick skin
Sour stomach

Dry, light, ribbony stools
Little sweating
Pearly white teeth
Tinnitus (ringing in ears)
Tonsillitis
Muscle tremors

Gastric ulcers
Uremia
Frequent urination
Varicose veins
Vincent's infection
Difficulty in focusing eyes

The Kelley literature also lists the following 'typical characteristics' of sympathetic metabolizers:

Like to make decisions
Actions usually explosive
Extremely active
Anger easily
Usually underweight
Rapid breathing
Irregular breathing
Eyes tend to protrude from sockets
Soles of feet soft and uncallused
Thin, flat chest
Face usually pale
Bowel movements normally light in color
Enhanced ability to concentrate
Crave sweets, fruits
Seldom depressed
Dislike fatty or oily foods
Weak dreams if any
Can't recall dreams
Seldom dream
A lot of 'get up and go' or drive
Dry hair
Dry skin

Ears very pale and light
Enjoy vegetables
Eating at bedtime interferes with sleep
Enjoy exercise
Thick eyebrows
Difficulty in falling asleep
Eyelids are opened wide
Strong emotions
Strong feelings of sexual passion
Fingernails have severe cross-ridges
Gag easily
Skin easily forms 'gooseflesh'
Dry mouth
Usually suffer from cold
Gums very pale or light
Severe indigestion
Impatient, irritable
Firm muscle tone
Pupils of eyes usually large
Violent reaction to unexpected noise
Thick, ropy saliva
Skin usually soft and velvety
Very jumpy and nervous

Your first reaction might be, 'Wow, I've a lot of those character-istics, I must be . . . ' Remember, these are *tendencies*, and to pinpoint the type as accurately as possible, Dr Kelley requires his patients to fill out a 3,200-item questionnaire and undergo an extensive blood test.

It is also wise to remember that a *balanced* metabolism may experience many of these characteristics or symptoms. Now, if *all* of those items on the list apply, you may be pretty certain you are a type 1, 4, or 6. You may also need a great deal of help.

Many of the listed terms went undefined. We did that on purpose. If you don't know what ketosis is, you probably don't have it. If you're curious, good for you — look it up.

Kelly comments on this group of metabolizers as follows:

Of these three, type 6 requires the most nutritional support, the greatest number and strength of vitamins, minerals and enzymes and other nutritional factors that help the vegetarian type. Type 1's require the second greatest nutritional support; they need the support that slows down the sympathetic nervous system and speeds up the parasympathetic. Type 4 metabolizers need the least nutritional support among these three — they are the closest to becoming balanced type metabolizers, and are fairly efficient metabolizers.

Kelley's research indicates the nutritional support most often needed by sympathetic-dominant metabolizers includes vitamins D, K, B_1, B_2, and B_6, ascorbic acid (vitamin C), biotin, folic acid, niacin, potassium, magnesium, zinc, chromium, hydrochloric acid, pancreatic enzymes, amino acids, and PABA. 'Each of the sympathetic dominant, vegetarian types needs these supplements,' he writes, 'but each type needs different amounts and different ratios. Sympathetic dominant metabolizers do *not* do well on high amounts of pantothenic acid, inositol, choline, lecithin and RNA supplements.'

Now let's look at Kelley's brief sketches of each of the three vegetarian types:

Type 1 metabolizers come the closest of all the types to being purely sympathetic dominant people. One of the chief characteristics of type 1 metabolizers is that they burn carbohydrates slowly. Their bodies use the carbohydrates poorly and they are able to maintain their blood sugar level with very little fluctuation. If anything, their blood sugar level stays a little elevated. With this condition, they can eat mostly fruits and vegetables, maintaining their health and feeling well. These people are what are commonly called vegetarians. They very seldom, if ever, crave meats (except fish) and when they eat meat, they usually feel groggy and have a loss of energy. These people do not do well on lamb, venison, beef, sardines or salmon. They can do quite well on up to 100% of their diet raw. They should stress the following foods: whole grains, including spaghetti, macaroni, breads, cereals, whole milk, eggs, white fish. They may use spices, 2-3 cups of coffee (non-instant), herbal tea, or an occasional alcoholic beverage or sweet dessert (made with unrefined sugar or honey). They enjoy and do well on nuts and seeds; rice, fruits and vegetables like apples, apricots, bananas, berries, grapes, oranges, pears, plums, grapefruit, asparagus, lima (butter) beans, beet tops, cucumbers, sprouts, lettuce, collards (cabbage), dandelion greens, kale, mustard, turnip greens, spinach and any leafy green vegetable.

Type 4 people are reported to have:

strong sympathetic nervous systems, but not nearly as strong as the type 1's. Type 4's are a little more balanced, or non-strict vegetarians. These people usually have a genetic background of their ancestors coming from around the Mediterranean Sea — Spanish, Italian, Greek, Israeli, Arabic, etc. Type 4's burn or metabolize their carbohydrates and sugars a little faster than the type 1's. The type 4's that tend toward having diabetes can normally control it with diet alone.

To maintain optimum health, type 4's do well on fish, chicken, turkey, other fowl, beef (twice a week), almost all vegetables, a little fruit, sprouts, some citrus, eggs and dairy products. Most American 'vegetarians' fall into this class. Type 4's generally need about 60% of their food raw. They normally do not need as much nutritional support in the form of nutritional supplements as do types 1 and 6.

A quick glance back at the metabolic type chart on page 40 will show you that type 3 is above the departure line from inefficiency of metabolism into efficiency, hence the tendency to need less supplementation.

Type 6, however, is below the efficiency departure line, even though headed back toward autonomic balance:

Type 6 metabolizers are people who are basically sympathetic dominant. They fall into the vegetarian class of metabolizers. Type 6's are very poor metabolizers — that is, they take in their food and nothing much happens. Their bodies do not utilize their food and they get very little energy from it and are generally sickly. Their assimilation or utilization of food is about 20% of normal. They almost always feel ill, or not up to par. Type 6's need about 60% of their food cooked. They need a great deal of supplemental nutritional support. They require more hydrocholoric acid, vitamins, minerals, enzymes, etc., than either Type 1 or 4.

Type 6 metabolizers should give care to the intake of whole and complete natural foods. All refined, processed, synthetic foods and additives must be avoided at all times. Type 6 people do best when they stress the following foods in their diets: adequate amounts of fruits and vegetables including lettuce, green vegetables, onions, radishes, potatoes; whole grains, including spaghetti, macaroni, breads; gelatin and other desserts made with honey; natural jams, jellies, ice cream, mushrooms, nuts, seeds, and seafoods and fowl, which should be preferred to other meats.

One's natural tendency here is to assume that particular types are 'bad' and that the object of nonspecific metabolic therapy is to move from a type 6 to a type 8 progressively. This isn't necessarily so. One objective of Kelly's program may be to improve the metabolism efficiency and seek a better balance between sympathetic and parasympathetic. However, genetics may play a key role in metabolism, so one's basic type may be fixed, or at least only partly improvable — if, indeed, 'improve' is the right word. A person can be a type 6 and function to a ripe old age. He or she will probably never feel 'terrific', but it doesn't necessarily hold that this person will die of cancer, arthritis, diabetes, or heart problems before turning forty.

Kelley's metabolic typing is an adjunct to the science and art of health and medicine — it allows the nutritionist and the physician to explore realms of probability heretofore overlooked or ignored altogether.

Sam, Carole's older son, was a maturing teenager when he started the Kelley program. His first typing was an 8 — balanced and efficient. As his body chemistry changed he tested out type 1, then type 4, and still later type 5. During that period his supplementation consisted of Kelley-program nutrition designed for each type. During the same period he experienced the enormous emotional stress of his father's death at roughly the same time he was graduated from high school and entered college. His Mediterranean heritage certainly played a key role in swinging his metabolism from balanced to sympathetic-dominant. The program surely played a role in bringing his near-total vegetarian metabolism back to type 4. His diagnosis as type 5 might seem mysterious until one learns he moved from Chicago to San Diego, utterly altering numerous environmental factors.

Jim, on the other hand, began as a meat eater, and except for a period of obvious fluctuation in his body chemistry during which a specific type could not be determined, he has remained a 5 balancing toward type 8, thanks to his mother's exceptional nutritional program.

Parasympathetic-Dominant Metabolizers: Types 2, 5, and 7

If you are a 'meat and potatoes' eater, you are undoubtedly curious about the parasympathetic-dominant type. Here's what Kelley has to say:

Group B metabolizers are classed types 2, 5 and 7. These types have very strong or dominant parasympathetic nervous systems. These parasympathetic metabolizers have strong function of the right brain, anterior medial hypothalamus . . . [and so forth — see Figure 3]. Their digestion is very good. They are not constipated, but to the contrary, they tend toward loose stools and diarrhea. They have poor muscle tone. They are in general lethargic, slow, fall asleep easily, but usually have a good reserve of strength and stamina.

Kelley's list of things the parasympathetic-dominant types are prone to include the following:

Craving for acid foods
Alcoholism (because alcohol raises blood sugar)
Alkalosis
Allergies
Excessive appetite
Arthritis (osteo, hypertrophic)
Asthenia (weakness)
Atherosclerosis
Asthma
Loss of control of bladder
Blackouts
Bloating
Low blood pressure
Easy bowel movements
Bone breaks
Brucellosis
Colds, flu, gripe
Cold sores, fever blisters
Mucous colitis
Chronic cough
Cough up mucus
Cramps
Dandruff
Dermatitis
Diarrhea

Fast, strong digestion
Diverticulosis
Drooling
Dropsy
Drowsiness
Eczema
Edema
Emphysema
Energy gain after eating
Energy loss after sweets
Chronic fatigue
Good fat metabolism
Foul-smelling gas
Gingivitis
Growling gut
Bleeding gums
Receding gums
oily hair
Hay fever
Headaches, eyestrain
Slow healing of bones
Massive heart attack
Hepatitis
Hernia
herpes simplex
Herpes zoster (shingles)
Hiccups

Histamine reactions
Hives
Hoarseness
Hydration
Hypoglycemia
Viral infections
Itermittent claudication
   (limping)
Jittery feeling
Leg ulcers
Leukemia
Leukopenia
Lymphoma
Melanoma
Nausea from eyestrain
Obesity
Osteoporosis
Periodontoclasia
Strong reaction to poison
   ivy, posion oak
Phlebitis

Good oxygen metabolism
Postnasal drip
Good protein metabolism
Psoriasis
Pyorrhea
Sexual problems, impotence
Itching skin
Sleepwalking
Sluggishness
Sneezing attacks
Stomach pain, excessive
   hydrochloric acid
Telangiectasis
Tingling in extremities (from
   deposits in vessels)
Duodenal ulcer
Urinary incontinence
Sudden urges to urinate
Ease in focusing eyes
Warts

And Kelley's list of parasympathetic-dominant characteristics goes on:

Extremely sluggish
Actions are relaxed, calm,
   firm, and positive
Desire to be cautious
Slow to make decisions
Above-normal appetie
Difficulty in holding urine
Bowel movements easy to
   start
Slow breathing rate
Frequently coughing up
   mucus
Frequent deep cough
Eyes look sunken in

Very enlarged, round chest
Ruddy complexion, good
   face color
Often feel sad or dejected
Very good digestion
Crave butter and fatty foods
   like cream sauce
Crave salty food
Crave fatty meats
Dream frequently
Dreams are vivid and often
   in color
Recall most dreams
Not much 'get up and go'

Oily skin
Pink or flushed ears
Feel better after eating at
   bedtime
Eating fruit causes jitteriness
Feel better and satisfied
   when eating meat
Emotional stability
Marked endurance
Intensely dislike exercise
Thin, scanty eyebrows
Droopy or saggy eyelids
Very little fear
Seldom get angry
Energy is elevated after eating

Face flushes easily
Fall asleep quickly
Orefer large egg-and-bacon
   breakfasts
Urinate several times
   a day
Gums dark pink or bluish
Excess saliva
Strong hunger pains
Intestines rumble and growl
   a lot
Eyestrain causes headache
Hard to get going in the
   morning

According to Kelly, metabolic types 2, 5, and 7 need some of the same nutritional support as vegetarian types, but for the most part they need entirely different vitamins, minerals, and foods to do well. Type 7, being below the efficiency departure line, needs more nutritional support than the other two carnivores, and the type 2 person is such a strong parasympathetic-dominant that he or she needs nearly as much supplemental support as type 7. Like type 4 on the vegetarian side, type 5 is more balanced and does not need as much supplement support.

The most often needed nutritional support for the parasympathetic trio includes Vitamins E and B_{12}, niacinamide, pantothenic acid, choline, inositol, calcium, phosphorus, calcium ascorbate, bioflavonoid complex, zinc, and RNA. Dr Kelley says that 'these metabolizers should eat at bedtime enough to carry them through the night. They should *not* eat leafy green vegetables, grains or cereals in great amount or take large quantities of the B vitamins. They generally do *not* do well on high amounts of ascorbic acid, niacin, potassium and Vitamins B_1, B_2 and B_6.'

By now, if you've been paying attention, you should be anticipating the obvious concerning the four balanced types,whose nutritional support we've yet to cover.

Kelly goes on to say:

Type 2's come the closest of all the types to being purely parasympathetic dominant. One of the chief characteristics of type 2 metabolizers is that they burn carbohydrates very rapidly. Their pancreases work so well that carbohydrates and sugars burn or metablize so rapidly that these people have a tendency to develop hypoglycemia — low blood sugar. When they eat only fruits, vegetables and sweets, their blood sugar rises and drops many times a day and their energy goes up and down like a yo-yo. When type 2's eat carbohydrates and sugars, they become very weak and shaky following a spurt of energy.

Type 2 metabolizers must have meat — preferably fatty, heavy, high purine meats such as lamb, beef, salmon, and sardines. They are usually the people that order their steaks very rare. By eating these fatty meats, they slow down their carbohydrate/sugar metabolisms. They feel they have eaten something that will 'stick to their ribs'. Their energy is released at a normal rate and they don't suffer the ups and down energywise that fruits and sweets cause them to experience. Normally, these metabolizers don't care much for sweets. They do well on root vegetables, cabbage, brussels sprouts, cauliflower, carrot juice and beans. They enjoy butter, cream, danish pastries, cream puffs and foods with cream or butter added. They can do well by adding a *small* amount of whole grains.

Type 2 people do very poorly on leafy green vegetables, candies, fruits, sweets, high carbohydrate diets and sugar pastries. They should limit the B vitamins and the intake of potassium supplements. Type 2 metabolizers usually have a genetic background from German, Scandinavian and Northern European ancestry.

Of the type 5 metabolizers, Kelley says:

They are persons who have strong parasympathetic nervous systems, but not nearly as strong as type 2 metabolizers. Type 5 metabolizers [tend] more toward the normal or balanced metabolism. They can tolerate a wide variety of foods. Type 5 metabolizers do well on beef or lamb several times a week; seafood, salmon, tuna, cheese, avocado, beans, peans, lentils, celery, carrots, asparagus, butter, whole grain cereals and breads, but not in great quantity, some nuts and occasionally danish pastry and cheesecake.

Type 5 metabolizers are not as prone to hypoglycemia as are the type 2 metabolizers. However, they can easily develop hypoglycemia if they indulge in too many candies and sweets. Many Americans fall into this class and do not do well as vegetarians.

The type 7 metabolizers are the sickly, weak parasympathetic-dominant class. They are inefficient metabolizers.

Their bodies do not utilize their food well and as a result, function very poorly. They almost always feel badly or sickly, functioning very sluggishly. It is difficult for them to maintain adequate nutrition to their individual body cells. Their body chemistry systems are quite inefficient and more than normal supplementation must be maintained at all times. Care must be given to the intake of whole and complete natural foods. All refined, processed, synthetic food and food additives must be avoided, constantly.

Type 7's are encouraged to stress the following foods in their diets: Seafoods, sardines, salmon, brains, liver, heart, meat gravies and soups; non-colored, unprocessed cheese, beans, lentils, carrots, celery, butter, cauliflower. Small amounts of danish pastries, cheesecake and an occasional alcoholic beverage may be taken. These 7's function best on purine meats such as salmon, tuna, beef, lamb and wild game. These meats should be preferred over others and used whenever possible and practical. Care should be given to adequately detoxify the bodies of these type 7 metabolizers.

Balanced Metabolizers: Types 3, 8, 9, and 10
The nutritional needs and characteristics of the more balanced types — 3, 8, 9, and 10 — may be anticipated by the careful reader.

Metabolizers in the balanced group have the greatest freedom in what they can eat. Indeed, they enjoy and thrive equally on foods from both the vegetarian and carnivore menus.

Kelley's research indicated that balanced metabolizers generally need nutritional support in the form of supplements including vitamins A, B_1, B_2, B_6, and B_{12}, niacinamide, vitamin C, bioflavonoids, vitamin E, folic acid, biotin, pantothenic acid, PABA, calcium, phosphorus, magnesium, manganese, chromium, and zinc. As was found in the other groupings, the amounts and ratios of the supplements vary among the four balanced types. Kelley has learned, however, that generally all the balanced metabolizers require extra amounts of hydrochloric acid and pancreatic enzymes. And these balanced metabolizers can suffer from the same conditions and disorders prevalent among either the sympathetic-dominant or parasympathetic-dominant. However, generally speaking the balanced group exhibits symptoms and characteristics in moderation and not to the extreme.

According to Kelley, balanced metabolizers are more prone to the following conditions:

Occasional acne
Normal appetite
Occasional asthma attacks
Normal blood pressure
Maintain normal weight
Normal cholesterol levels
Occasional cold sores or
    fever blisters
Normal blood sugar
Seldom have diarrhea
Fairly good digestion
Occasional hiccups
Normal pulse rate
Catch cold occasionally
Occasional infections
Occasional itching skin
Occasional sweating
Occasionally has coated
    tongue

Occasional sour stomach
Occasional stomach ache
Seldom have spells of
    sneezing
Normal skin texture
Normal reactions to insect
    bites
Seldom get motion sickness
Occasional rash or hives
Occasional nausea
Seldom have insomnia
Occasional indigestion
Occasional rumbling of
    intestines
Occasional headache from
    eyestrain
Hay fever once in while
Occasional emotional upset

Some of the typical characteristics of the balanced metabolizer are as follows:

Actions are occasionally explosive
Normal alertness
Occasionally get angry
Occasional periods of fatigue
Sometimes experience belching
Normal bowel movements
Eyes are set normally in sockets
Normal thickening on soles of feet
Average-size chest
Face color is normal, not pale or flushed
Like a wide variety of foods
Sometimes have dreams
Have a fair amount of drive
Hair is not too oily, not too dry
Skin is not too oily, not too dry
Like to eat fruit, but also like meat
Normal endurance
Eyelids — eye slits, normal (lids not drooping)
Fall asleep within a reasonable length of time
Normal amount of sexual passion
Don't mind exercise when time is available
Gums have normal color tone — not too light or too pink
Seldom have hoarseness
Don't get hungry between meals
Have coffee occasionally
Normal initiative and energy
Normal stools, neither hard or loose
Very seldom need laxatives
Get started in morning without too much trouble
Occasionally cough up mucus
Once in a while do things on impulse
Sometimes have a sense of ill health
Eyes have very little sensitivity to strong light
Like all kinds of salad dressings
Saliva is normal, not too thick or thin

Occasionally need extra sleep
Occasional splitting of nails
Seldom if ever have mood changes
Handle stress fairly well
Voices are normal, not low- or high-pitched
Don't worry much
Normal-size bowl movements
Skin is not too thick, not too thin
Occasionally have reaction to shots or injections
Can tolerate quite a bit of pain
Don't get excited easily
Stable but occasionally run out of energy

Well, you might say, that list sounds pretty normal. And well it should! However, the word 'normal' is so often vague as to be specious. Were you to line people up along the sidewalk and ask a group of people to select the ones most 'normal', you would be amazed at the diverse reasoning — notwithstanding the influences of the electronic media on stereotyped thinking.

Summary
Before moving on, let's summarize the metabolic types.

Group A
Type 1 — Strong sympathetic dominance, close to being purely vegetarian. Very slow oxidizers of carbohydrates. Cannot do well on red meats or other high-purine-content protein foods such as salmon or sardine. Type 1's do very well, however, on a 100 per cent raw diet.

Type 4 — Moderately strong sympathetic dominance, but tending toward balance. Slightly faster oxidizers of carbohydrates than type 1. Won't be made to feel ill, weak, or queasy by red meats, but require, and desire, very little. Does well on 60 per cent raw food.

Type 6 — Moderately sympathetic dominance, but very inefficient metabolizers. Require a great deal of supplementation suited to their vegetarian bent. Need about 60 per cent of their food cooked and cannot cope well with processed, denatured foods. Require supplemental hydrocholric acid to aid digestion.

Group B

Type 2 — Strongly parasympathetic dominance, a first-order carnivore. Fast oxidizing system, perhaps too fast, tending to hypoglycemia. Cannot do well on fruits and vegetables as energy level acts like a yo-yo. Large meat meals are quite satisfying, especially fatty, heavy, high-purine meats. The stereotypical 'steak and potatoes' person.

Type 5 — Moderately strong parasympathetic dominance tending toward balanced metabolism. Tolerate a wide variety of foods, but many develop a tendency toward hypoglycemia and cannot do well as a vegetarian.

Type 7 — Moderate parasympathetic dominance, tending to move away from balance, but at the same time an inefficient metabolizer. Sluggish and sickly much of the time. May do better if they stress organ meats such as brain, liver, heart and high-purine muscle meats. Refined, denatured foods wreack havoc with the inefficient metabolizer. Care needs to be taken to detoxify these types.

Group C (Balanced)

Type 3 — Balanced autonomic nervous system, but the worst metabolic efficiency possible. Do not do well at all in modern environment because of assimilation problems. Require excellent-quality natural foods of a wide variety and good amounts as well as strong nutritional supplementation.

Type 8 — The most common type found among Americans who are reasonably healthy. Good, well-balanced autonomic system, better than average metabolism efficiency. Able to survive fast food and supermarket fare better than most because of autonomic system's adaptibility and efficiency. Not superman, however.

Type 9 — Balanced and only slightly below the line of departure into inefficiency of metabolism. Cooked food is demanded and a very wide variety of foods seems the best support.

Type 10 — Uncommonly efficient metabolizers who seem to get abundant use of their food, hence don't need large amounts. Energetic, can eat almost anything and do well, but seem to prefer fruit, vegetables, whole grains, and cheese.

There we have the Kelley thesis. Now, how about his proof? How did Kelley come to these conclusions? Do his conclusions withstand scrutiny? Let us see in the next chapter.

Chapter Five:

How the Kelley Program Works

Ours is a dynamic universe in which things are constantly changing, and the metabolic types are no exception. They are neither constant nor static; metabolic processes ebb and flow in response to a myriad environmental influences, notably nutrition. Dr Kelley's problem was to find a way to capture the dynamism of metabolism, nutrition, and individual types in some meaningful, economical, understandable program.

Enter the computer. Without computer technology, the procedures required for the Kelley Metabolic Ecology program would be so time-consuming as to be priced totally out of usefulness. Painstaking diagnostics and analysis, like those which caused the economic demise of homoeopathy (the prime form of medicine prior to 1900), threatened Kelley's methodology before it started.

To computerize metabolic typing, Kelley and his researchers assigned numbers to metabolic function, with 1,000 standing for excellent health. In this way he designated an individual's 'metabolic index', which he demonstrates to be the estimated summary of the nutritional condition of a particular person. The numbers are derived from the responses to the 3,200 questions the individual must answer about his health and life-style, and from Kelley's particular methods for scoring the results of blood and urine tests.

Once a Kelley physician has all the data on a patient, the carefully programmed computer takes over. In the scale of 0 to 1,000 the number 700 is considered 'normal' and 600 'low-normal', so it is desirable to score above 700 or, ideally, in the 800s.

Each individual on the program receives a printout of his or her nutritional program. This volume, generally called the Kelley Book, is a combination of individual data printed by the computer and general data on nutrition and detoxification and basics, including natural food recipes, that fills 136 pages. Persons who are serious about achieving optimum health, or who are very ill and have opted for the Kelley program, will usually be reevaluated every six months.

Carole and her sons, who are nothing but numbers to the computer, can look back over their programs for the last several years and see the changes — not necessarily improvements in every case, however. For example, the stress of the death of Carole's first husband, the boys' father, evidenced itself in the programs following the event. Each of us lives in a constantly changing environment and our reactions to the constant change affect our health.

In one of the programs, back in 1981, the printout section of Carole's book describing her metabolic index reads: 'Areas below 600 should be carefully observed. They may have escaped your attention because they are not pathological. Although these areas are not clinical, there is a real need for your attention and consideration. With this early warning system, you can make prevention a more realistic part of your practice. If, on the third or a subsequent evaluation, an area remains low, or even becomes lower, in addition to the nutritional program, your special attention, energies, knowledge and clinical application should be utilized.'

Now, that's obviously a general-program statement suited to every person. In the beginning of their programs, Carole, Sam, and Jim observed many numbers on their metabolic index that bore asterisks and listed below 700, some even below 600. Like many others, they were coming to the Metabolic Ecology program with all the atrocious eating habits of the supermarket culture. Carole insisted that all three of them adhere to the nutritional programs that their Kelley 'Books' outlined for them. All three improved considerably toward more optimum health. They are not optimum at this point, but then it takes time to restore health to bodies that have been unhealthy for many years.

If you go on the Kelley program for a quick fix, you will surely be disappointed. Physicians dispensing drugs in allopathic practice provide the quick fixes; that's their specialty. The nutritional approach may occasionally surprise many people with its efficiency and speed of improvement, but it's designed to maintain balance and prevent degeneration, and rebuild body function, naturally. It's not an overnight remedy.

Carole's 1981 metabolic index listed her as a 'functional metabolic type 8, and a sub-type 1'. Figure 5 (page 71) is a reproduction of Carole's computerized evaluation. As you can see, she is quite 'normal'. The largest number, 20200, is under the designation for 'type 8'. The second largest number is under 'type 1' (pure vegetarian) — 17675. Hence her subtype grouping. You may have noticed that under the major categories — 'Sympathetic, Balanced, and Parasympathetic' at the top of the chart — Carole's numbers indicate she leans much more toward vegetarianism than meat eating. Nothing wrong with that, although the Kelley program aims individuals, always, towards balance. The 'Developmental Type Chart' numbers reflect what Carole's type was during childhood and puberty. Unlike many people tested, Carole's type as an adult is not the direct opposite of her type during youth.

In the columns reproduced from Carole's metabolic index (Figure 6), she was delighted to see only two asterisks — for liver and muscle development. They signified potential trouble spots, or the weakest links in her metabolic system. Were this some form of generalized data bank, those two lower evaluations would be meaningless. However, in Carole's individualized program, both aspects were significant. Therein lies the strength of the individual metabolic evaluation. Your chart will make sense to you, for you, and about you.

How accurate is the Kelley evaluation, you may wonder? In our household it withstood the challenge of time and scrutiny and we are convinced that it proved to be the best health-giving program we could have adopted.

There have been very few detractors from among the thousands and thousands of chronically ill patients who stuck with the Kelley program for a reasonable length of time, and most of the detraction, which we discuss later, is not technical or scientific; it's economic or personal preference.

Now, to get a better perspective on metabolic types altogether, this is a good place to quote Dr Kelley at length on the subject of his theory behind the development of metabolic types, research problems he faced, and the phenomenon of changing metabolic types.

The development of Metabolic Types can be best appreciated from an evolutionary perspective. We would suggest that originally the forerunners of the human species displayed a balanced type of metabolism, ideally suited to a hunter-gatherer lifestyle. These prehistorical humans evolving in a temperate ecosystem would have had access to a wide variety of vegetable foods, nuts, seeds, occasional meats and fish. A flexible physiology, capable of utilizing a variety of foodstuffs, would have most definitely been an evolutionary advantage.

Interestingly, Kelley's thinking itself evidently evolved to an evolutionary viewpoint, which holds that diverse physical characteristics come about as part of a 'natural evolutionary process.' However, how the differences within species came to be isn't nearly as important to us right now as the recognition that differences do exist. The human body has managed to adapt to tremendously diverse environments, so obviously the metabolic system comes with a built-in adaptability factor, whether the theory of evolution is correct or not.

Continuing his explanations, Kelley says:

However, during the past fifty thousand years, climatic conditions throughout the earth have hardly been stable, and enormous adaptive pressures would have been in operation. Particularly, during the last ice age some thirty thousand years ago, many of the earth's temperate regions — once hosting a rich and varied flora and fauna — would have converted to either tundra-like ecosystems or, at equatorial latitudes, desert systems due to the great amount of water tied up in the ice ranges. In either case, ecosystems reverted to more stressed, less diverse states. And these climatic changes exerted great selective pressures on our prehistoric forefathers. Our ancestors who chose to remain in the colder regions could have survived only if they carried the genetic ability to utilize meat as the predominant component of their diet, since the extreme cold diminished the availability of plant food sources. Eskimos, who traditionally hunted animal foods before the advent of civilized produce in their territory, might be seen as the modern day descendants of these hardy, cold-enduring ancestors. Eskimos have for ages subsisted and in fact thrived on virtually all-meat diets — certainly an extreme aberration from the temperate climate diet of the original balanced metabolizers.

On the other hand, other descendants of the original balanced humans most probably migrated into more desert and temperate regions around the equator. Here, vegetable foods, nuts and seeds would have been the most readily available foodstuff, and only those humans with the genetic makeup to thrive on such foods would have survived. Hence, we have the ecological conditions ripe for the selection of sympathetic dominant vegetarian type humans, who would have had little need for a physiology adapted to a meat oriented diet.

Of course, this is an oversimplification, but it is important to realize the important role the genetic variability has played, even within historic times. For example, a sympathetic dominant type physiologic makeup would have been necessary for the first agrarians settling in the rich Middle Eastern floodplains some ten thousand years ago. Such peoples subsisted largely on a grain-based diet, including only occasional meat proteins and milk proteins. These agriculturalists could in fact only have survived with a predominant sympathetic genetic makeup. On the other hand, the ancestors of the North American Plains Indians, for example, living in a temperate climate notable for a rich and varied animal life population, thrived as nomadic hunters. Such peoples would have survived only if natural selection had allowed for the development of a predominant meat-eating physiology; otherwise human life would very quickly have ceased on the great American Plains.

Each individual is born with a certain type of metabolism. One can only do himself harm by ignoring his metabolic type and basing his diet on a particular whim, philosophy, or religion, rather than the genetically-determined needs of his own body. One should recognize his or her metabolic type and live in accordance with it. It is extremely difficult for an individual to make a change in his basic metabolic type. The understanding and application of this concept is imperative and a very significant part of one's individualized metabolic program.

In researching the metabolic types of modern Americans, Kelley encountered a number of research problems. First, the available literature indicated that serious studies were made only between the turn of this century and 1930. These studies were limited to certain laboratory animals and certain cultural groups such as Italians, Germans, Swiss, and Norwegians. Additionally, these early studies concluded that metabolism is a fixed inherited factor and cannot be changed. No classification of types was made, although the early researchers occasionally noted things that did not agree with clinical findings and simply dubbed them 'anomalies' without further explanation.

Again, Kelley's problem was to collect data, explain them, and devise a way to make them useful. Many of the earlier 'anomalies' are explained by metabolic typing.

Kelley goes on to explain:

Everyone is aware that America is the melting pot of the world. This is quite true in regard to the metabolic types. All types of people of different nationalities, cultures, religions, and so forth have intermarried until there are almost no true or pure 100% metabolic types in our society. There is such a mixture of these genetic factors that it has been very difficult to develop the metabolic classification. As more data was collected, it was learned that one person could have certain dominant characteristics from several metabolic types. Through modern research, it is now possible to determine to what extent an individual's metabolism is functioning from each of the different types.

It became known that certain factors do influence the metabolic type within which an individual is functioning. Classification has been refined to the point where it is possible to determine in percentages how a person is functioning in each of the 10 metabolic classes.

In other words, a person might function as follows: as a type 1, 15 per cent; a type 2, 1 per cent; a type 3, 4 per cent; a type 4, 33 per cent; a type 5, 3 per cent; a type 6, 11 per cent; a type 7, 6 per cent; a type 8, 12 per cent; a type 9, 7 per cent, and type 10, 8 per cent. Kelley then adds:

When individuals were re-evaluated, it was found that they had flipped metabolic types; that is, they now had an entirely different percentage rating on their tests. After much more data collecting and after innumerable calculations were combined with new research, it became possible to formulate additional conclusions. Essentially, the following took place:

Up until the early 1900s, the ethnic and culture groups in our society were fairly stable. Their metabolic patterns were constant and in general would stay the same throughout a person's lifetime. By the early 1940s the mixing of genetic backgrounds became so complex that very few, if any, metabolic patterns were of a true and pure type. This gave rise to the percentage mixtures of the metabolic types.

Then, by the 1950s, medical science had achieved low infant mortality rates, giving rise to high incidences of the defective metabolic types 3, 6 and 7. By the early 1960s, the stress of modern life-styles was causing severe exhaustion of genetic metabolic dominant types.

For example, a person with a strong genetic sympathetic nervous system dominance has excellent function of the left brain, anterior pituitary, parathyroid, thyroid and adrenal medulla glands; heart, bone, muscle and connective tissue, kidneys, gonads (ovaries or testes), and uterus or prostate. Eventually, the stress of the life-style begins to exhaust these glands and organs, causing the person to feel bad. His life-style stresses his sympathetic glands to total exhaustion. He now has only his weaker parasympathetic nervous system glands with which to maintain life. He becomes lethargic and depressed and starts going from doctor to doctor to no avail. He tries to maintain his life-style, causing exhaustion of his parasympathetic glandular system. When this occurs, the person flips into a type 6 metabolism. With even further exhaustion, he flips into a type 7. And with still more exhaustion, he finally becomes metabolic type 3 and his system is so inefficient he is not capable of coping with what is considered routine by healthy individuals.

Another example would be a person who has a strong parasympathetic nervous system. He is a happy, calm, 'nothing makes me mad' type of person. He is slow but powerful and has a lot of reserve and enjoys life. In trying to keep up a rapid pace, he exhausts his parasympathetic system. Consequently he flips into sympathetic dominance and becomes irritable and high strung, gets insomnia and becomes a strange new beast at home and work. No one has the slightest idea what is wrong. He now puts pressure on his weaker sympathetic system and it collapses under the strain. He then flips into a type 7. He finally flips into type 3 like his original opposite in the first example. His health is in deep trouble and he must make adequate changes immediately.

Another factor entered the picture by the late 1960s and early 1970s. Agribusiness has been responsible for the production of food consumed in our nation, and people have become more interested in taste and eye-appealing factors than in the intrinsic nutritional factors. Our foods have been hybridized and chemicalized beyond normalcies. Consequently, poor nutrition is now a major stress on our metabolic processes.

The Kelley program was designed to deal with the many variables of the living body, especially the 'flips' our bodies make from one metabolic type into another while we are journeying from chronic complaining to excellent health. In 1984, years of research by Kelley's long-time assistant, William L. Wolcott, culminated in an additional set of metabolic factors being included in the Kelley program.

Time after time metabolic therapists encountered symptoms and reactions in their patients that strayed from the carefully calculated metabolic-typing molds. Years of intense probing finally uncovered the culprit — oxidation rate. The next chapter deals with Wolcott's research and conclusions.

Figure 5. Sample metabolic type evaluation.

Metabolic Type Evaluation

D0590   03/02/81-06   643-4536-6   1313231

Functional Type Chart

Sympathetic		Balanced		Parasympathetic
40.96		33.33		25.69
		Type 10		
		3030		
		3.22		

Type 01	Type 04	Type 08	Type 05	Type 02
17675	16665	20200	13433	9090
18.81	17.74	21.50	14.30	9.67
	Type 06	Type 09	Type 07	
	4141	7070	1616	
	4.40	7.52	1.72	
		Type 03		
		1011		
		1.07		

The above chart shows your metabolic type to be 08
and your metabolic subtype to be 01.

Developmental Type Chart

Type	1	4	6	3	8	9	10	7	5	2
Score	1111	404	1818		4444	4141	2020		2121	707

From this chart your developmental type is 08
and your developmental subtype is 09.

Figure 6. Sample metabolic index.

Balanced		Sympathetic	
General Metabolism	819	Heart	830
Acid/Alkaline Bal.	821	Circulation	778
Autonomic Nerv. Syst.	812	Blood Vessels	809
Centr. Nerv. Syst.	792	Memory	789
Glandular Bal.	835	Skin	838
Hormone Balance	846	Stress Sensitivity	767
		Thyroid Gland	838
Parasympathetic		Parathyroid Glands	813
		Calcium	882
Immune System	789	Phosphorus	832
Thymus Gland	827	Bone System	848
Lymph System	850	Red Blood Cells	821
Bone Marrow	839	Drive or Motivation	782
White Blood Cells	746	Pituitary Gland	801
Saliva Glands	781	Adrenal System	831
Lungs	867	Genitourinary	812
Hemoglobin (Iron)	818	Muscle Nutrition	810
Cell Protein	822	Muscle Development	656*
Protein Metabolism	825	Magnesium	842
Pancreas	792	Potassium	887
Carbohydrate Metabol	822	Sodium Chloride	851
Zinc	839	Kidneys	803
Assimilation	827	Cranio-Sacral Mech.	845
Elimination/Colon	806	Dental Structure	820
Hydrochloric Acid	791	Neck Vertebra	829
Mineral Metabolism	835	Upper Back Vertebra	829
Vitamin Metabolism	796	Lower Back Vertebra	828
Enzyme Efficiency	800	Connect Tissue Sys.	880
Liver	727*	Ligament Development	848
Fat Metabolism	823		
Cholesterol	841		

Functional Metabolic Type   8

Chapter Six:

Fast, Slow, and Mixed Oxidizers

In the first chapter we cited Dr George Watson of the University of Southern California for his original contribution to the studies of metabolic individuality. Dr Watson wrote *Nutrition and Your Mind* (Bantam, 1972), wherein he explained in understandable language how the oxidation rate works within our bodies. Watson was a psychologist, so his primary interest centered on the relationship of oxidation to emotional and mental characteristics. Other researchers attempted to follow up on Dr Watson's research but encountered difficulty in duplicating his results with consistency. Wolcott and Kelley point out that the researchers who failed probably did not take the autonomic nervous system dominance into consideration.

Oxidation is the process of turning nutrients into energy. Carbohydrates, sugars and starches, proteins, and fats are all metabolized in our cells in two principle energy-forming stages. These stages are known as (1) glycolysis and (2) the Krebs cycle, or citric acid cycle. Glycolysis consists of nine steps, the Krebs cycle of eight steps. There are specific mineral and vitamin requirements for every step of the two-stage process and if certain requirements are missing or lacking because of improper diet or improper supplementation, the entire oxidative process may be fouled up and the body may suffer an energy shortage.

As a result of the successful completion of the two oxidative stages, 100 per cent of the body's potential energy becomes available. However — and this is crucial — the successful completion of the Krebs cycle depends upon the successful completion of glycolysis. Dr Watson wrote that the terms 'fast oxidation' and 'slow oxidation' refer mainly to glycolysis. To be technical, yet simplistic, the perfect process requires an exact amount of oxaloacetic acid, which is a by-product of glycolysis, to combine with acetyl coenzyme A. Oxaloacetic acid is extracted from carbohydrates, while acetyl coenzyme A is taken from proteins, fats, and carbohydrates.

Therefore, Watson and Wolcott agree that, in Watson's words, glycolysis 'ultimately regulates both the rate of energy release and the amount of energy that may be formed.' Wolcott stresses:

Both fast and slow oxidation result in inefficient energy production from the oxidative process, but for virtually opposite reasons. In the slow oxidizer, there exists in the body adequate or even excess acetyl coenzyme A, but carbohydrates are burned too slowly, producing deficient quantities of oxaloacetic acid from pyruvate. Therefore, in the slow oxidizer, there is insufficient oxaloacetic acid formed to convert acetyle coenzyme A into energy in the Krebs cycle.

Conversely, the fast oxidizer burns carbohydrates far too quickly and in too great a quantity in glycolysis, producing an excess of oxaloacetic acid. Unfortunately, the fast oxidizer is also deficient in acetyl coenzyme A production and therefore, like the slow oxidizer, does not have the capacity for full energy production from oxidation. Both the fast and slow oxidizers have the same problem: the inability to adequately utilize acetyl coenzyme A in the Krebs cycle. Whereas the fast oxidizer is not producing enough acetyl coenzyme A, the slow oxidizer who produces enough can't turn it into energy.

Now, how does this fit in with metabolic typing?

Wolcott noted that in metabolic typing a sympathetic-dominant person is normally viewed as a slow oxidizer and a parasympathetic-dominant person as a fast oxidizer. However, clinical evidence analyzed by Wolcott for several years showed clearly that sympathetic-dominants who are also fast oxidizers and parasympathetic-dominants who are slow oxidizers do, indeed, exist — and drive therapists crazy! 'Sympathetic fast and parasympathetic slow', Wolcott reported,

account for a smaller percentage of the population when compared to the sympathetic slow-parasympathetic fast, and this smaller segment of the population has its own set of unique biochemical patterns and requirements. The balanced autonomic type can also be a fast or slow oxidizer. And theoretically, there can also be a balanced oxidizer who is either sympathetic, parasympathetic or balanced in autonomic function. However, it would be extremely rare to achieve and maintain a perfectly balanced oxidation rate, although one could closely approach balanced oxidation given the proper balance of biochemical support.

As you can imagine, the concepts of fast and slow oxidation out of synch with the metabolic type caused consternation, to say the least. Competent metabolic therapists were running into serious complications. In fact, two examples taken from Wolcott's detailed research paper allow us to explain in practical terms what this is all about.

Wolcott lists them as 'example 1' and 'example 2'. I prefer the more vivid fictional designations Long Tall Sally and Short Fat Suzy.

Long Tall Sally is middle-aged, and her chronic complaints center on tension and anxiety. She's what many of us would call 'high strung'. She was unable to shut her mind off at night, suffered from insomnia, nervousness, fretfulness, and recurring high blood pressure. She felt 'hyper'. Her complexion was pale and she tended to be underweight. She talked rapidly in a nervous-sounding voice. However, she started the Kelley program as a 'normal' type 8 — relatively efficient and balanced. She moved into a type 4 program and was on the 4 program when Wolcott entered the act. Long Tall Sally was a good patient, she followed the program explicitly and faithfully, but still she fidgeted and fussed and remained high strung. Wolcott wrote:

Her technician evaluated her properly and in accordance with the metabolic type model, but felt that she was probably too sympathetic and too acid, so he suggested moving to a type 1 diet instead of a type 4. Normally by stimulating the parasympathetic system more strongly and increasing the intake of more alkaline foods, such symptoms are alleviated. However, these changes produced instead a slight worsening of the symptoms.

Next, the technician, still believing the symptoms to be indicating acidosis and sympathetic dominance, increased her potassium intake, changed her type formula from that of a type 4 to a type 1, and increased her B vitamins. This alteration along with a type 1 diet produced a definite worsening of the symptoms.

Long Tall Sally was probably ready to chuck the Kelley program onto the quack heap and go back to martinis and cigarettes. After all, everything they tried by the book on her individual metabolism made her feel worse. Her body reacted in a way that was diametrically opposite to what was anticipated. Stay tuned for the exciting conclusion of Long Tall Sally's metabolic perils.

Short Fat Suzy was in her mid-twenties, and from all the classic metabolic typing she was parasympathetic-dominant. She started out on a type 5 program, then went to a type 8, then a type 2, and finally back to type 5. Poor Suzy, she didn't have any serious medical complaints that an allopathic doctor could get excited about, but she complained of fatigue, depression, loss of memory, lack of motivation, low sex drive, obesity, bloating, and listlessness.

Wolcott wrote: 'She reported noticeable improvement on the first program. She also apparently did well on the second program. By the middle of the third program, however, she reported feeling as though her original problems might be returning. By the fourth program, she definitely felt the presence of her old problems and felt as though she had made no progress at all.'

Like Long Tall Sally, Short Fat Suzy had been a faithful patient, taking all her supplements and doing her detoxification by the book. Also like Sally, Suzy had nothing in her environment that could be construed as a cause of her problem: no trauma or emotional upset, for example. Wolcott went on:

Believing the woman to be too parasympathetic, the technician restricted even more the fruit and vegetable intake. This, again, had the opposite effect — it seemed to take away her energy even more. At that point the technician increased the adrenal support and increased the Ultra Cal and Calcitrate [calcium supplementations] and doubled the type 5 formula. This procedure again was in total accord with the model. Surprisingly, this last recommendation caused a noticeable and definite worsening of the patient's symptoms.

Obviously these were extraordinary, rare case histories, but it is the forte of Kelley's metabolic typing system to deal with every unique individual. The two cases could not be ignored and turned away as 'anomalies', which is standard procedure throughout much of medical practice. What actually happened and what was learned from the experiences?

Long Tall Sally was most definitely what the Kelley metabolic typing system calls an 'inefficient sympathetic'. Though she may have exhibited a few classic symptoms of sympathetic dominance, her reactions to a highly parasympathetic alternative indicated she was most certainly not a classic sympathetic type. 'Normally, giving potassium and B vitamins to a sympathetic will have a calming, sedating effect due to the biochemical effect of stimulating the parasympathetic system', Wolcott noted. 'But in this case, these nutrients had the opposite effect. This was because those nutrients had a stronger impact on increasing the oxidation rate than on the innervation of the parasympathetic system.' So it was discovered that Sally not only had a relatively strong sympathetic-autonomic dominance, but also had developed an increasingly fast oxidation rate. This combination served to bolster hyperactivity on several levels and wound up manifesting, in her case, what appeared to be symptoms of classic sympathetic dominance.

When it was determined that Sally was apparently a fast oxidizer rather than a normal sympathetic slow oxidizer, the physician took her off the type 1 formula and put her on a type 2 (extreme parasympathetic) diet along with calcium supplementation and a type 5 (more balanced parasympathetic) formula. 'Her B vitamins were decreased as well, and the results were dramatic,' Wolcott reported. 'Within hours, her symptoms showed definite improvement which continued through the weeks following the change in program. The changes that were affected pertained, in this case, primarily to the oxidation rate rather than the autonomic type.'

Short Fat Suzy, on the opposite side of the autonomic spectrum, had all the physical traits, mental and emotional characteristics, personality, and adverse symptoms to mark her clearly parasympathetic-dominant. No metabolic technician worth his salt would have listed anything about her as sympathetic-dominant. But, as in Sally's case, when the physician tried to treat her with classic parasympathetic-dominant procedures, she became worse. 'What actually occurred,' Wolcott said, 'was that instead of affecting the sympathetic autonomic function in the anticipated manner, the supplements and diet pushed her body chemistry into severe slow oxidation.'

Once again the result was exactly the opposite of what the physician had learned to expect. 'In her case, however, it was not necessary to reverse her supplemental program. Changing to a type 4 diet and adding magnesium, potassium and some B vitamins was all that was required. The results were quick and dramatic. By changing her program to a more parasympatheticizing program, this woman actually lost her adverse symptoms and began to demonstrate some sympathetic qualities, such as more energy and motivation, improved memory, no depression and a more positive outlook for the future.'

Wolcott, who is working with me on a major book tentatively titled *The Physiology of Behaviour*, observed some key facts about metabolic types and oxidation rates:

The influence of the autonomic nervous system indicated by the autonomic types, sympathetic and parasympathetic, is a primary cause for, and the basis of, physiological characteristics that one may be prone to, and also certain psychological characteristics. Oxidation rate appears to relate primarily to qualities stemming from the energy or lack of energy produced through the oxidative process. Most definitely they have an influence on most all physical, mental and emotional symptoms, although they may not be of primary cause.

Speaking in the most general terms, the qualities of slow oxidation (hypoactivity, depression, alkalinity) most closely parallel those of parasympathetic-dominance. Those of fast oxidation (hyperactivity, anxiety, acidity) parallel those of sympathetic-dominance. Thus, we see a natural balance, a dynamic interrelationship between autonomic function and oxidation rate where the autonomic type and oxidation type work in complementary fashion with each other, forming a dynamic balance in the healthy person. Each appears to work upon the other in a push-pull, check-and-balance type of situation. Whereas the influence of the autonomic nervous system stems essentially from the brain and the hypothalamus, or, if you will, the mind, the influence of the oxidation rate on metabolic characteristics stems from intracellular activity, the body. Certainly there are synergistic relationships involved, but this model is useful in explaining many cause-and-effect relationships between the mind and the body.

Wolcott points out that normally the abundant energy associated with sympathetic dominance is counterbalanced by a slower oxidation rate, cutting back on the hyper or 'push' tendencies. Speed up that oxidation rate somewhat and the hyper tendencies may become adverse symptoms, and a strong sympathetic-dominant (high-strung vegetarian) with a fast oxidation rate could have real problems.

Another aspect to consider, according to Wolcott, is the acid-alkaline balance. Sympathetic dominance tends to produce acidity. The stronger the sympathetic dominance, the greater the potential for high acidity from the greater yield of metabolic by-products. Slow oxidation tends to produce alkalinity, so once again we have strong evidence of the ongoing dynamic balancing interrelationship.

Normally in a healthy sympathetic-dominant, the autonomic function is slightly stronger than the oxidation rate. Therefore the sympathetic tends to be energetic and slightly acid. But, if a sympathetic develops fast oxidation, a strong propensity for problems of acidity and severe metabolic imbalance are developed because both sympathetic autonomic function and fast oxidation tend to produce acidity rather than alkalinity.

The parasympathetic-dominant derives energy primarily from a fast oxidation rate since the sympathetic neuro-endocrine function is usually weak in parasympathetic dominance. As in the case of the sympathetic, the oxidation rate normally serves to balance the strong parasympathetic tendency toward alkalinity. Fast oxidation is acidic, thereby balancing parasympathetic-dominant characteristics, but whenever the oxidation rate slows down, producing alkaline-type qualities, the individual will be affected adversely.

Wolcott summed it up as follows: 'Whereas the autonomic balance may play a primary role in the existence of the myriad characteristics of the metabolic type, the oxidation rate can enhance, support, overshadow or even negate the autonomic based symptoms.'

Wolcott's research indicates that while the metabolic-type determinations based upon autonomic functions may aid physicians in tracing the primary causes of degenerative disease, oxidation rate should not be viewed as a primary cause for physical traits, individual anatomical characteristics, or efficiency levels of organs, glands, and systems. For example, a degenerative trend involving calcium deficiency (which is quite common) could be due to biochemical imbalances found in either fast *or* slow oxidation.

> A fast oxidizer has an actual deficiency; and a slow oxidizer has an intracellular calcium deficiency due to the lack of . . . synergistic factors necessary for calcium utilization. The oxidation rate influences the quality and rate of energy release from cellular oxidation of glucose, which in turn flavors or shades or gives rise to different qualities of energy levels, personality, and so forth. It would probably be more accurate to say that the particular mineral/vitamin balance or imbalance gives rise to the oxidation rate as well as determining particular tendencies of a degenerative nature, rather than to say that the oxidation rate is responsible.

That rather technical discussion boils down to the idea that the oxidation rate most strongly affects energy levels, personality traits, and reactions to foods. This fine distinction becomes important when you are taking vitamin and mineral supplementation in the hope of improving your health. Wolcott pointed out that 'normally' the kind of nutrients that stimulate or increase sympathetic dominance also increase or cause a slower oxidation rate. Conversely, the supplements that 'normally' stimulate parasympathetic dominance also stimulate faster oxidation rate.

A key factor that Wolcott discovered was that

supplements and diet which increase the slow oxidation rate *always* increase slow oxidation, and likewise for supplements to increase fast oxidation rate. However, critically, the supplements and diet which usually bring about sympathetic dominance do *not* always do so; likewise for parasympathetic supplementation. Whether certain supplements or diet affect autonomic dominance as anticipated depends on the state of metabolic balance between the autonomic types and the oxidation rate at the time of administration.

To make this point clear, and to give us a lesson in nutritional science, Wolcott turned to the research of Dr Watson. According to Watson, the following list of nutrients will assist the breakdown of carbohydrates to oxaloacetic acid in glycolysis, which means these supplements would increase the oxidation rate and push the individual from slow to faster oxidation.

vitamin B_1	vitamin D
vitamin B_2	potassium
vitamin B_6	magnesium
PABA (para-aminobenzoic acid)	copper
niacin	manganese
ascorbic acid (vitamin C)	iron

At the same time we are to note that these same supplements would normally be considered parasympatheticizing according to the Kelley model. However, this is correct only for classic sympathetic slow oxidizers. They would play hell with a sympathetic or normal parasympathetic fast oxidizer, but they could be helpful to a parasympathetic slow oxidizer if the effects of the oxidation rate outweighed that of the parasympathetic autonomic function. We'll learn why this is shortly, but first Watson's list of nutrients that bring about a slowing of the oxidation rate:

vitamin A	vitamin C
vitamin E	bioflavonoids
vitamin B_{12}	zinc
niacinamide	calcium pantothenate
choline	phosphorus
inositol	iodine
calcium	

Again, these supplements are used in the Kelley model to be sympatheticizing — the kind of nutrients one would take to balance a parasympathetic dominance.

Now, before we continue this exploration in nutritional science, think about all the thousands of poor souls who march into health-food stores or vitamin shops with fists full of money and zero knowledge. Does the shopkeeper or clerk know all this about oxidation rates and individual metabolism? What do you think? No wonder the establishment maintains a dim view of the health-food and vitamin retailing business.

On the other hand, some of the storekeepers must have hit it right with some of the customers — the people keep coming back for more. Is it luck? Or is it wishful thinking in the guise of positive attitude? Think about this. The shotgun approach to vitamins and mineral supplements we take in the marketplace may actually be doing more harm than good. How many times have we heard someone remark, 'Well, even if it doesn't help, it can't hurt.' Au contraire!

Every vitamin and mineral has specific synergistic or blocking relationships with other vitamins, minerals, and chemicals in the body. 'In terms of the effect on autonomic types and oxidation rate,' Wolcott reported,

> the two most important minerals are calcium and potassium. Calcium works synergistically with magnesium and in opposition to potassium and sodium. As intracellular calcium and magnesium levels go up, intracellular potassium and sodium levels tend to go down. Conversely, as potassium and sodium levels go up, calcium and magnesium tend to drop.
> In terms of oxidation rate, intracellular calcium levels tend

to rise in slow oxidation and fall in fast oxidation; potassium tends to be lower in slow oxidation and high in fast oxidation.

Kelley's metabolic-typing procedures utilize the metabolism of calcium in determining a person's autonomic dominance, among other things. The normal sympathetic-dominant (slow oxidizer) has good calcium metabolism with adequate to excess calcium, a factor also seen in slow oxidation. Conversely, the normal para-sympathetic-dominant tends toward poor calcium metabolism and is usually prone to calcium deficiency, which also goes along with fast oxidization.

Thus we can see that what is truly one man's meat may be another's poison. The Kelley program strives to bring us from dominance of one part of the autonomic system toward balance. In the process there will be instances where the individual's oxidation rate will be at cross-purposes with the program, or at least the program won't suit the oxidation rate at all.

Like vitamin and mineral supplementation, selection of food plays a significant role in manipulating or adjusting metabolic type and oxidation rate. The same features are present as for the vitamin-mineral supplementation, however. Foods that tend to increase parasympathetic dominance also speed up the oxidation rate, and conversely those foods that increase sympathetic dominance also slow down oxidation rate. Foods that cause speeding up or slowing down of oxidation rate always do so, but those foods designed to stimulate either sympathetic or parasympathetic dominance are not so consistent; they do the job depending upon the metabolic type in question.

Wolcott gives an oxidizing diet in brief as follows:

Eat liberally of low fat, low purine protein such as eggs, fish, chicken, turkey and some nuts; all fruits and their juices, all vegetables and their juices, especially leafy greens; all grains and cereals. Restrict or eliminate butter, oils, fatty meats, and dairy products.

The slow oxidizer does not do well on fats. Fats are known to bind magnesium, preventing efficient calcium utilization, allowing intracellular calcium levels to rise, resulting in slow oxidation. The slow oxidizer also has sufficient quantities of acetyl coenzyme A, of which fat is a major source, but lacks oxaloacetic acid, which is derived from carbohydrates. The slow oxidizer is usually a sympathetic dominant and sympathetics usually don't have the digestive capacity to adequately handle fats. Fruits and vegetables are a high source of potassium, which is vital to increase the oxidation of carbohydrates in glycolysis. Dairy products are often high in fat and usually high in calcium and low in magnesium, which is necessary for proper calcium utilization. The slow oxidizer already has excess calcium, so more isn't needed; rather the need is for synergistic factors to help calcium utilization.

As for the opposite side of the coin, the diet for the fast oxidizer would consist of the following:

Fatty, high purine meats and all meats are acceptable; dairy products; root vegetables, barley and corn meal plus fats, nuts, oils, butter and cream.

The fast oxidizer should restrict or eliminate all grains except barley and corn meal, almost all fruits and leafy vegetables. Unlike the slow oxidizer, the fast oxidizer does well on fat, in fact needs to eat fat. The fast oxidizer is deficient in acetyl coenzyme A, and fats provide a major source. Usually, the fast oxidizer is also parasympathetic-dominant, and normally has the digestive capacity to easily accommodate fats and high purine proteins. By allowing calcium levels to elevate, fats help slow the oxidation rate down. However, most grains, due to their high phytate [phytic acid] content, tend to lower the calcium levels in the body, which exacerbates the already existing calcium deficiency of a fast oxidizer.

Fruit and leafy vegetables, being high in potassium, also worsen the mineral imbalance of a fast oxidizer by again lowering calcium while contributing to the existing higher levels of potassium. Dairy products provide high levels of both calcium and fat, both of which are desperately needed by the fast oxidizer. Calcium not only helps slow the oxidation rate, it acts as a stimulant to the sympathetic system at the same time.

Wolcott has learned from clinical experience which dominant influence — autonomic or oxidative — is the basis for the symptoms being exhibited by the individual. However, out here in the dining rooms of the world we may not be so discriminating.

'Eat your salad — it's good for you,' is a common parental imperative. Well, maybe that salad isn't good for the fast-oxidizing little chap, and maybe Mother doesn't know best. Just maybe!

It seems to me that many of us will 'crave' those foods our system needs as if by instinct. Then again, I've heard some experts say that a person may crave things that are detrimental (foods that he is allergic to, for example). What would that phenomenon be? Instinctive death wish?

It all comes down to how much we do not know as opposed to how much we think we know. A cynic once said, 'Ignorance isn't the problem; it's so many people knowing so many facts that ain't true.'

Wolcott's research into the autonomic dominance and oxidation rates led him to examine one of the most dreaded diseases of modern times — obesity. I have a bit of a problem with my weight, so the following information caught my attention:

> The tendency for overweight problems is usually relegated to the parasympathetic dominant, but it also occurs in the sympathetic dominant as well. Two examples of different types of obesity in terms of the metabolic type model may clarify the issue.

Wolcott sites the first example as a 'classic overweight parasympathetic':

> This woman was 50 years old, 5'4" tall and weighed 204 pounds. She had tried many diets to lose weight, all ending in dismal failure. Most had involved low fat, low protein regimes. This was the reverse of what she needed. As a fast oxidizer, she burned her carbohydrates too rapidly and did not have enough acetyl coenzyme A from fat and protein to combine with the excess levels of oxaloacetic acid from the carbohydrates. The diet simply made things worse.

When she started a type 2 program (designed for meat eating parasympathetics) to push her toward sympathetic slow and having a balancing effect, she lost seven pounds in one week, and her diet consisted almost wholly of meat, butter, oils, cream, dairy products and some vegetables. Her problem was her need to balance her oxidation rate, allowing her to burn the calories she took in more efficiently.

Wolcott then cites a second example, another obese woman, only this time a sympathetic, very slow oxidizer:

Whenever she ate fats and oils she immediately gained five to seven pounds. Whenever she avoided such foods, she lost the excess weight and more. By eating fats, she greatly exacerbated her already slow oxidation rate, which disallowed her oxidative process to efficiently burn the acetyl coenzyme A from fats. She could eat just about all the carbohydrate she wanted and do nothing but improve her oxidation situation.

In the case of the latter individual, Nathan Pritikin would have a definite winner and Dr Atkins a loser.

Wolcott's specialty in the area of metabolic research is in the area of the physical effects on psychology. He offered some interesting observations in that regard as well:

How is it that a sympathetic-dominant can feel slowed down, tired, exhausted, without an obvious strenuous cause? It is the sympathetic autonomic function that is responsible for the left brain dominance, rational mental sharpness, good memory, quick recall and so forth. Sometimes these qualities in a sympathetic may diminish, weaken or slow down without actually losing sympathetic dominance. When this occurs it is due to the oxidation rate going too slow. At such times, giving potassium can actually restore sympathetic strength rather than generate a shift into parasympathetic dominance.

Usually, the brain appears to reflect most quickly any shifts in oxidation rate. Often, one may observe what seems to be clear mind/body splits in terms of symptoms, which can be easily understood with this metabolic type model. For example, a young woman reported that at times her body would feel really fast but her mind would feel really slow. She also discovered at such times that drinking lemon juice seemed to balance her out.

What actually occurred was a result of her being in a state of sympathetic slow. Her autonomic function was felt in her body and the slow oxidation rate in her mind. The lemon juice was an excellent form of potassium. Taking the potassium stimulated her parasympathetic system, tending to balance her sympathetic dominance and at the same time it served to increase her oxidation rate, restoring liveliness to her mind.

The Kelley model presumes that depression is most commonly found in persons who are parasympathetic-dominant and slightly fast-oxidizing types. However, it can occur and be equally devastating with a sympathetic, extremely slow oxidizer. Wolcoll sites this example:

At 11.30 p.m. a call was received by a 61 year old man. He was crying uncontrollably and in his words was 'suicidal'. He had been typed as a parasympathetic fast and was on a strong program to push him toward sympathetic slow, which involved a lot of meat, fatty foods and calcium. Learning that he had followed his program to the letter, but had also been under tremendous physical and emotional stress, the obvious interpretation was that he must have gone into severely slow oxidation. It was recommended that he take ½ teaspoon of cream of tartar dissolved in a glass of water.

Remarkably, within 20 minutes he called back and sounded completely normal. His spirits were up and he even told a joke and laughed. This case is an example of how potent and powerful food and nutritional supplementation can be. Many times, just stopping the wrong diet or supplements can provide a tremendous increase in well-being, and even a little of the right food or nutritional substance can provide a tremendous change in biochemistry.

The cream of tartar was an excellent, quickly assimilable form of potassium. Ingestion of the proper nutrients for one's metabolic type should produce favorable results quickly. If they do not, then, in all likelihood, the wrong recommendation has been given.

Finally, to evaluate people's oxidation rates in general terms, Wolcott prepared the following questionnaire. The kind of oxidation rate indicated by each trait is given in parentheses following the answers.

1. Physically I feel most of the time:
a. exhausted (slow)
b. speedy (fast)
c. tired (slow)
d. hyper (fast)
e. speedy but exhausted (fast)
f. energetic (fast)
g. energy goes up and down (fast)

2. Appetite:
a. strong most of the time (fast)
b. poor most of the time (slow)
c. mostly strong, sometimes not (fast)
d. need to eat often to feel at best (fast)
e. no desire for breakfast (slow)
f. wake up at night hungry (fast)
g. need to eat before sleep to sleep well (fast)

3. Memory:
a. diminishing capacity (slow)
b. excellent (fast)
c. poor after eating a heavy meal (slow)
d. better after eating fat (fast)
e. poor after eating just fruit or cereal for breakfast (fast)

4. Ability to have strong thoughts and carry through to a conclusion:
a. good usually (fast)
b. poor usually (slow)
c. almost always can do that (fast)
d. often feel mentally groggy or slow (slow)

5. For main meals I usually or normally prefer ——.
    (Answer not what you think you should have, but what you
    would like to have if it were okay.)
a. something light — salad, chicken or fish (slow)
b. an accompanying dessert (slow)
c. something heavy to stick to the ribs (fast)
d. substantial food like meat and potatoes (fast)
e. ample butter, ample salt (fast)

6. For breakfast, I feel better an hour or so later if I eat:
a. a heavy breakfast (fast)
b. a light breakfast (slow)
c. an abundant meal (fast)
d. little or nothing (slow)
e. some kind of meat included, steak, bacon (fast)
f. just some cereal, maybe with some egg (slow)
g. just a little fruit or juice (slow)

7. I love to eat, or prefer to eat:
a. sour-tasting foods (fast)
b. sweets and desserts (slow)
c. fruits (slow)
d. salty foods (fast)
e. fatty foods (fast)
f. red meat (fast)
g. white fish (slow)
h. potatoes (fast)
i. rice or green salad (slow)

8. If I'm tired, eating a meal:
a. makes me sluggish (slow)
b. makes me energetic (fast)

9. If I'm tired and I eat something sweet:
a. I feel less tired, with more energy that lasts (slow)
b. at first, I feel a lift, then I seem to become tired again, sometimes
    more than before (fast)

10. Breakfast:
a. I can often skip it and do fine until noon (slow)
b. I need to eat or by midmorning I'm very hungry and exhausted
    (fast)

11. Between meals:
a. I can get a voracious appetite (fast)
b. I rarely think of food or eat snacks (slow)

12. Lunch:
a. If I don't eat a heavy lunch, I tend to lose my energy by midafternoon (fast)
b. If I eat a heavy lunch, I become sleepy an hour or so later (slow)

13. After supper:
a. I would just as well have buttered, salty popcorn as a sweet dessert (fast)
b. I feel more satisfied if I have a sweet dessert (slow)

14. If I believed that butter was good for me, and not harmful (as claimed by margarine-industry propaganda):
a. I would eat it a lot (fast)
b. I still would eat it very little (slow)

15. Sweet foods such as desserts and candy:
a. I often enjoy them and they seem to make me feel fine (slow)
b. They taste too sweet to me (fast)

16. Going for four hours without eating:
a. often leaves me exhausted, hungry and sometimes irritable (fast)
b. causes no ill effects (slow)

17. Eating a heavy meal in the evening:
a. perks me up (fast)
b. sometimes leaves me depressed (slow)
c. restores my energy (fast)
d. makes me tired and sleepy (slow)

You may have discovered that, according to this test, you're pretty well mixed up — at least that's how I scored. One time I'm fast, the next time I'm displaying aspects of a slow oxidation rate. If you experienced the same mixture of answers, consider yourself fairly normal. Like the type 8 metabolizer, you are probably balanced and reasonably efficient in oxidation rate as well as autonomic nervous system.

Of course, a simple quiz like this is not meant to give a definite diagnosis. For persons with chronic symptoms who have spent small fortunes on medical doctors to no real avail, a visit to a qualified Kelley metabolic therapist may prove exceptionally helpful. The Kelley program has been upgraded to include all the latest research involving oxidation rate. (Kelley has said that he has learned from his studies of metabolism and health never to be dogmatic. He promises to keep learning and upgrading and changing.)

Finally, in an attempt to summarize the combined interrelationship of oxidation rate and autonomic dominance, Wolcott states:

True good health is a state of homeostasis. It is one in which all the body organs, glands and systems function efficiently in a state of dynamic equilibrium. Everything is relative to each individual's inherent metabolic design limits. Theoretically, health can be seen in a sympathetic-dominant person, a parasympathetic-dominant, a very fast oxidizer, a slow oxidizer, as well as in the balanced autonomic and oxidative types.

The key lies in how the autonomic type relates to the oxidative rate. If they exist in a state of dynamic equilibrium, health is indeed probable. A sympathetic type 1, sub-type 4, with a very slow oxidation rate can conceptually be as healthy as a slightly sympathetic type 4, sub-type 5, slightly slow oxidizer. However, it is recognized that the former would be more restricted to the sympathetic qualities while the latter would have not only access to sympathetic qualities, but also greater access to parasympathetic qualities. Though they differ in capacities, each individual could live a healthy, productive life within the individual design limits.

It is when the dynamic equilibrium is lost between autonomic type and oxidation rate that health is considerably diminished and there exists the potentiality for the development of adverse symptoms. One might expect problems in a slightly sympathetic, extremely slow; a very sympathetic fast; a parasympathetic extremely fast or a very parasympathetic extremely slow and so forth.

Together, the autonomic type and the oxidation rate determine the overall metabolic type and define the requirements of nutritional individuality. It is imperative for the practicing nutritional therapist to accurately determine their interrelationship. It is only in so doing that the therapist will be rewarded with success. If the requirements of the nutritional individuality are correctly fulfilled, the results can be so astonishing as to appear to stem from a realm of magic. It is only then that the therapist can understand from his own experience that truly, food can be our medicine or our poison.

Chapter Seven:

Learning to Eat Right for Your Type

If you sign on with the Kelley Metabolic Ecology program and receive the Kelley Book that contains your personal computerized program, you will read in the introduction this brief summary of the Kelley approach to health:

The human body is made up of approximately one hundred trillion cells. These cells are constantly metabolizing the nutrients supplied to them. By the time you have read this sentence, over one million, three hundred fifty thousand cells will be born in your body replacing those that no longer function efficiently. One billion new cells are made each hour. Each cell in itself is far more complicated than even the most intricate electronic computer, and all the cells together form the most complex system that can be imagined — your body.

We know of and have isolated about 50 nutritional substances which the body must have regularly to maintain growth, development and a normal healthful condition. In addition, there are numerous unidentified substances in natural foods which are known to be of value. The human body is the most complex and intricate chemical laboratory ever designed. It takes in the air we breathe, the water we drink, the food we eat and through millions of biochemical and bioelectrical reactions, produces a beautiful life force — YOU. And there can be only ONE you.

You are unique as is every human being. Each of us is different from one another in every facet of our being: genetic design limits; structural characteristics; external physical characteristics; size, shape, placement and efficiency of each of the bodily organs, glands and systems; rate and efficiency of metabolism; blood chemistry; psychological characteristics and personality traits. The natural result of our metabolic individuality is our nutritional individuality — the need for differing kinds, amounts and combinations of nutrients and raw materials to sustain our metabolic life processes.

The Kelley Book goes on for 136 pages in which it details the individual's program and outlines general practices to make the program work effectively. The metabolic program proves to be extremely complicated from the research point of view, but it boils down nicely and is easy to understand.

Kelley was asked in an interview, 'Does this concept ever seem unscientific to you?' His response was:

Not at all. To me it's more scientific than conventional or crisis medicine, because it entails knowing the reasons for malfunctions of the body. If you've mastered physiology, biochemistry, biology and nutrition, you're going to be able to effectively help the body to actually recover from the imbalances that are causing the symptoms. To me that's a lot more scientific than suppressing a symptom with a powerful drug, then letting the patient go home and wait for his body to heal itself. It isn't that we don't understand how to deal with specific organs or systems when they reach a stage of breakdown, it's that we know if you isolate just one organ and treat it, chemical imbalances will merely shift and the problem will crop up later in some other form.

The Kelley program was scientifically designed to do the following:

- Review the nutrients in your present diet, pointing out certain shortages, excesses, and balances.
- Suggest foods that will provide nutrients that may be deficient in your present diet.
- Recommend the necessary food supplements to replenish the nutrients that may be exhausted in your body.

- Balance your dietary intake of proteins, carbohydrates, fats, oils, vitamins, minerals, enzymes, intrinsic factors, calories, and so forth.
- Instruct you in basic principles of cleansing your body in order to eliminate the many toxic substances that may have accumulated owing to environmental factors, faulty diet, improper nutrition, and inefficient elimination.
- Utilize your foods, supplements, vitamins, minerals, enzymes, etc., in the most efficient manner possible.
- Point out the physiological reactions your body may have as it receives the optimum nutritional factors.
- Instruct you in the basic principles of good nutrition and a healthful life-style.
- Explain the proper and most helpful diet for your individual needs.
- Explain ways of preparing food that conserve nutritional values.
- Provide sample menus to serve as a guide to correct food preparation for your individual metabolic requirements.
- Present recipes for nourishing, whole, natural, health-giving foods.
- List helpful sources of information that one can study and build 'a whole new life of healthful living'.

No wonder it took twenty years to put this program together! Kelley and his researchers studied food preparation in painstaking detail, taking pages from numerous health authorities, in order to list recipes and menus and tell how foods should be prepared. For example, the Kelley Book even tells the reader how best to boil an egg.

Did that statement pique your curiosity? In fact, the entire report on eggs is so interesting and detailed that we'd like to reprint it here to illustrate the depth of study that went into the general dietary instructions of the Kelley Book.

Eggs are an unusually good source of protein. They are well balanced and the standard by which all protein is evaluated. They have all the essential amino acids in proper proportions.

Many of us have been incorrectly taught to use only the yolk of an egg. But it is best to use the whole foods, and a whole egg is both yolk and white. Both parts are needed to complete the digestive pattern of an egg. It's true that the yolk contains natural lecithin and may be considered as a source of natural fat.

Eggs should always be chosen from hens that are naturally raised — on the ground, and with roosters. It is important that the buyer check to see that the chickens are fed on grains without antibiotics or other drugs, and that greens, earthworms and insects are available to them. (Similar rules apply to duck eggs, which have far more protein and are a much better buy than hen eggs if they are available.) It is a MUST that only the best eggs be used. If none but the chemicalized, devitalized eggs sold in grocery stores are to be found, it will be far better to do without eggs completely.

Proper preparation of eggs is of vital importance. The egg must be heated in the shell at a temperature of 140 degrees to 160 degrees F (the normal temperature of really hot tap water) for five minutes before it is cracked. This destroys an enzyme just inside the membrane under the shell that prevents the biotin in the egg from functioning normally. When biotin functions properly, it greatly reduces the cholesterol risk of eating eggs.

After preheating the eggs before cracking them, they may be fixed and eaten in any way desired. Soft boiled and raw eggs are the most preferable, though it isn't absolutely necessary to eat them in those forms. In keeping with the use of as much raw food as possible, a good procedure is to eat the eggs raw in a blended drink of some kind, flavored to suit one's taste.

There was a group of research doctors and dentists who, for at least a dozen years, had eaten two eggs daily (properly prepared as above), as a part of a well-balanced nutritional program. Tests conducted on these people showed no increase in cholesterol. In fact, there was a significant decrease in the blood serum cholesterol level of each individual.

Misconceived beliefs of the orthodox medical world about eating cholesterol-containing foods have caused countless people to be unduly alarmed about cholesterol levels and the associated possibility of heart attacks. These misconceptions, carried on from the early 1950s, have been proved false.

As you can see, the Kelley Book can be eye-opening. Oh, yes, the part about boiling an egg properly is found later in the book. The recipe says to put a quart of water in a deep pan and bring it to a boil. Slip the room-temperature eggs in carefully so they don't crack, cover the pan, and reheat the water to a boil, but only for a few seconds. Then remove the pan from the heat, keep it covered, and let it stand until the water is cool, or about twenty-five minutes.

Let us warn you that not all the suggestions in the Kelley Book are necessarily appetizing. For example, read this: 'Liver is a wonderful energy food and cannot be surpassed as a blood builder. *Raw* liver contains enzymes and amino acids which are destroyed when it is cooked, and it seemingly has other beneficial factors. Comparative tests of people eating raw liver and cooked liver show differences that science has not yet fully explained. There are no supplements or drugs that can take the place of raw liver; none are in any way comparable in their effects.

Although it presents authoritative and interesting information about nutrition — appetizing or otherwise — the Kelley Book also acknowledges the limits of nutrition. Kelley points out that 'a passenger car is not designed to haul gravel — a gravel truck is not designed to be an ambulance. Men are not designed to have babies — women are not designed to have hair on their chests. Each individual must learn the limits of his or her design and capacities. The very best nutrition can do no more than help maintain physiological function within the individual's design limits.'

While Kelley has proved conclusively that proper nutrition for the metabolic type indeed prevents and allows the body to fight or resist many chronic deficiency conditions, including cancer, he stresses that 'Nutrition cannot rebuild a birth-defected body. Nutrition cannot redevelop missing tissue, replace needed surgical operations, substitute for structural adjustments, meet the needs of psychological counselling, fill cavities or correct all disease conditions.'

He follows that with his potent message of hope: 'Proper nutrition can, and does, prevent, lessen and help heal the chronic deficiency conditions that plague our society. Good nutrition is absolutely necessary to help prevent birth defects, chronic diseases, delinquency, crime, senility, exhaustion, depression and the multitude of other conditions that are so persistent.'

Under the heading 'Suggested Nutritional Supplementation', the book becomes downright personal. Following a couple of pages of general information on food supplements, your computerized data match supplementation to the specifics from your answers to the 3,200 questions and what was deduced from your blood and urine analyses. We deal with the subject in depth in the forthcoming *Nutritional Supplements*.

A major segment of the Kelley Book is devoted to 'detoxification', which we cover in the next chapter. Then comes 'Physiological Reactions to a Well Balanced Nutritional Program'. In this section Kelley tells the reader what to expect.

As you follow a properly balanced nutritional program, changes begin to happen within your body. Often this is alarming and not at all what you expected to happen.

The ideal reaction is the gradual development of an increased 'sense of well-being'. At first you will notice you do not tire so easily. You 'last' longer during the day, and you do not become tired so early in the evening. Next, you find you are not so tired in the mornings. You look forward to the new day and may awaken earlier. As your sense of well-being increases, you begin to feel more emotionally and psychologically secure. Little things do not bother you as they once did. Your old habit patterns begin to change from 'grumpy' ones to 'happy' ones.

The ideal reaction often occurs, but more frequently there is a multitude of uncomfortable reactions which normally come first as your body chemistry begins to change. These reactions should not alarm you or cause undue apprehension. Any one or all of the following reactions may occur:

After about two or three weeks on this program, it is normal to experience toxic reactions. You will gradually lose your appetite, become nauseated and may even develop a 'toxic headache'. Occasionally, you may also experience swelling in the various lymph glands throughout your body. These toxic reactions are brought about by the normal cells cleaning debris from the system faster than the liver, kidneys, skin and lungs can remove them from the body. At this point you can do two things to help:

1. Discontinue the supplements for no more than a five-day period. Continue the supplements again for ten days. This cycle of five days off and ten or more days on may have to be repeated several times, depending upon the depleted condition of your body and the amount of repair which is needed at the cellular level.

2. Take a coffee enema to stimulate the excretion of toxins. The procedure for this is explained earlier in the program. One or two a day may be taken depending upon the severity of the toxic condition. In an extreme toxic reaction, both the discontinuance of supplements and the coffee enemas should be used.

Sometimes you may experience an allergic reaction. This is particularly true when the hydrochloric acid in the stomach is deficient and/or when the liver and adrenal glands are in a state of disfunction or extreme exhaustion. The allergic reaction is similar to the toxic condition. You may just not feel well, be nauseated and/or even develop a skin rash, shortness of breath, etc. This can be brought about by taking too many supplements at once for the first time. If you tend to be allergic, you should start your supplemental program by taking only one supplement for three days, then adding the second one. Continue both for three more days, then add the third supplement. In three days, add the next one and so forth, until you can tolerate the complete suggested supplemental program.

As you begin to physiologically balance your body chemistry, other reactions may take place. It is not easy to change from lifelong habits of faulty eating of devitalized, processed foods to a new system of eating natural, life-giving foods and taking individualized needed supplements.

Following this metabolic program should bring about a readjustment of body chemistry. The body, meeting this changing situation, often responds in surprising ways to this process. The longer the deficiencies have existed, the more prevalent the response is likely to be. Additional reactions may occur as the body adapts and stabilizes. The reactions that often occur are: excessive gas, migrating pains, rash or hives, running nose, headaches, insomnia, increased thirst, weakness, loss of appetite, nausea, diarrhea, fever blisters, dry mouth, canker sores, constipation, nightmares, dizziness, nervousness, craving unusual foods, and various body aches and pains, both in the joints and muscles. When these reactions occur, you can be assured your body is responding and changes are taking place. If you think of these as correcting crises, it will be easy to accept them as steps on the road to better health. If they occur, they are only temporary and are but a small price to pay for the long-lasting benefits.

You might be thinking, 'Ha, that's easy for him to say!' However, remember that Kelley himself went through the agonies he describes, when he cleansed his own system and created a nutritional program to save himself from terminal pancreas cancer.

Carole, Sam, and Jim experienced almost all of these adverse reactions when they started the program several years ago. Not all at once, of course, but during the process one or the other of our family experienced just about every named symptom.

Generally speaking, we are most of us pretty much creatures of bad habits, and we may find it hard to accept the withdrawal symptoms on top of having to swallow all that strange stuff that's so good for us. However, as Kelley said, it's a small price to pay for good health.

Chapter Eight:

Cleansing Your System for Better Health

In the begining of his program book Dr Kelley points out that the human body is made of something like 70 to 100 trillion cells — a quantity impossible to conceive of. Why, the American national debt is only around one to two trillion, and even that amount is unimaginable!

Even more mind-boggling, perhaps, is the realization that each of our 70 to 100 trillion little garbage receptacles needs dumping out regularly. Unfortunately, as Kelley points out, our technically advanced society, despite all its 'experts', has not really understood the proper procedures for cleaning up this multitude of garbage-laden cells.

Most of us go blithely along, sipping carbonated sugar-water, munching oversweetened or oversalty snacks, dining on refined hydrogenated, chemicalized, additivized, denatured meals, drinking unbelievably bad water made worse with chemicals such as fluoride and chlorine, breathing polluted air, wandering past flora dripping with poison sprays, coating our skin with chemicals that make us look and smell 'better' — and in short, keeping those trillions of garbage cans stuffed and overflowing.

Eventually the miracle of our human body is exhausted and the garbage begins to win. We feel lousy and begin showing the symptoms of myriad chronic disease. Ain't life wonderful? Our kids are born in worse shape than we were ever in at that age, and we probably started off with various and sundry problems due to our parents' crummy habits, ad infinitum. The Kelley program attacks the problem head on. It's not exactly painless, but it's proved effective and far less painful and expensive than the alternative of disease.

A cleansing program is not to be undertaken casually. During the process, the cellular metabolism is speeded up, and the bloodstream and organs of elimination might not be able to cope with the load. Kelley's program is designed to moderate each individual's detoxification to prevent toxemia. Cancer patients, Kelley explained, have been known to die from the sudden release of too much toxin into the system after going on a detoxification program. Their bodies are riddled with toxins as a result of the disease, and then the toxic load is increased by radiation or chemotherapy treatments.

Once a change in nutrition begins to take hold, the toxins just naturally want out. It's this sudden flood of garbage that accounts for the various symptoms Kelley warned of in the previous chapter.

You've already learned that digested food is absorbed into the blood and lymphatic systems to be assimilated by the cells. Your digested food, along with oxygen, is transferred into your cells, which cells metabolize everything. Every cellular metabolic process results in waste-garbage. The process of eliminating this waste is every bit as vital to life and health as the process of digestion.

The accumulation of waste is poison, no matter which metabolic type you are. Kelley's program does its best to help you deal with elimination of the excesses accumulated over the years.

'As the cells produce metabolic debris', Kelley's book stresses

the blood carries it to the organs of detoxification. These organs are the liver, kidneys, lungs, skin, many of the mucous membranes, and the colon. If these organs of detoxification are themselves filled with debris, they of course cannot accept further debris from the cells and, before long, there are 70 to 100 trillion garbage cans completely full. It is like the city dump being filled to capacity and not accepting any more garbage trucks. Then one's home becomes overloaded with garbage, which shortly interferes with normal functions of one's household. Before long the entire community has become bogged down. 'Clean blood', then, acting as a highway for the garbage trucks, is dependent upon the organs of detoxification.

Kelly explains that the liver is the major area of detoxification and also the organ that is most stressed by our modern life-style.

The liver's job is to separate out metabolic wastes as well as chemical pollutants and other contaminants in our food, and to eliminate them. It is the liver that keeps the heart healthy — not to mention the kidneys, the pancreas, and the brain. Our society is reverently concerned with the health of the heart but ignores the importance of the liver. You don't see many 'liver foundations' springing up, do you?

People worry about their livers generally after the onset of hepatitis, cirrhosis (generally from too much alcohol), or infectious mononucleosis. Of course it's a little late at that point, but then human nature is like that. Kelley goes on to list all the substances we've been decrying throughout this book — substances that place 'undue stress on the liver'. We repeat the list, in case you missed it:

chemicals of any kind; drugs; synthetic foods; artificial food additives such as coloring, preservatives, emulsifiers, stabilizers, sweeteners, etc. [including the very popular MSG or monosodium glutimate chefs love to use]; alcoholic beverages; carbonated beverages; hair sprays; chemical deodorants; and reheated vegetable oils used in frying, etc. Unrefined oils, or butter for sautéeing, can be used without creating peroxides and free radicals which are toxic to the liver.

If more people realized what the liver does for them, they wouldn't be so cruel to it! The liver has to metabolize essential fats like cholesterol, tryglycerides, and lipoproteins in order to keep them from running amok in the bloodstream, where they may form deposits on arterial walls. The liver must synthesize the bulk of necessary blood proteins for the body's use. It's responsible for breaking down and eliminating *most* drugs and environmental poisons. Nature produces a lot of toxins, so primitive humans had to have good liver function. However, nature's relatively few toxins are nothing next to our manmade stuff.

The liver manufactures and secretes bile, and bile is the cellular garbage man. No bile, no elimination. And if you can't eliminate, you die! If that's not enough, bile also acts essentially in the digestion and assimilation of all fat-soluble nutrients. This amazing fluid takes from the blood the worn-out hemoglobin with its attendant waste, which gives feces its brown coloration.

Kelley notes that today a tremendous number of people, including teenagers, fail to have

free, unobstructed flow of bile from the liver and gall-bladder in response to the food entering the small intestine. Eating refined or processed foods, eating fresh food which is mineral deficient because it is grown on depleted or chemically treated soil, lack of regular vigorous exercise, stress, multiple distractions during meals, and many other unnatural aspects of our lifestyle have combined to alter the chemistry of bile so that formation of solid particles from bile components is a commonplace occurrence among Americans. These solid particles remain in the gall-bladder or the base of the liver for many years and become progressively harder, sometimes calcifying into 'gallstones'. Long before this occurs, however, metabolic problems are under way. When a significant number of solid bile particles accumulate, the free flow of gall-bladder contents is diminished, causing progressive stagnation and congestion of the liver. The body begins to suffer the effects of poor assimilation of fat-soluble nutrients, which may play a role in the development of eczema, psoriasis, dry skin, falling hair, tendonitis, night blindness, accumulation of calcium in tissues, and sometimes prostate enlargement in men. Hemorrhoids and varicose veins draining to the liver are often the result of this congestion.

The Kelley program devotes a great deal of attention to cleansing the liver with liver and gall-bladder 'flushes', a technique that Kelley says he borrowed from the world-famous Lahey Clinic Medical Center in Boston, Massachusetts.

Kelley prefaces the instructions for such flushes with: 'The importance of cleansing the debris from the liver and gall-bladder, thus keeping the bile free-flowing, cannot be overemphasized.' There are four basic, active principles in the procedure:

1 — Apple juice, which is high in malic acid, or orthophosphoric acid, which acts as a solvent in the bile to weaken adhesions between solid globules.

2 — Epsom salt (magnesium sulfate), taken by mouth and enema, which allows magnesium to be absorbed into the

bloodstream, relaxing smooth muscles. Large solid particles which otherwise might create spasms are able to pass through a relaxed bile duct.

3 — Olive oil or other unrefined oil, which stimulates the gall-bladder and bile duct to contract powerfully, thus expelling solid particles kept in storage for years.

4 — Coffee enemas, which consist of a coffee solution retained in the colon. They activate the liver to secrete its waste into the bile, enhancing bile flow and further relaxing the bile duct muscle.

Kelley stresses that these flushes are an important procedure for persons over fifteen years of age, and he suggests that patients seek their doctor's approval (good luck!) so that they can repeat the flush every two months.

Now, if you want to flush out, please write to the International Health Institute (see page 134 for address) for literature and talk it over with your doctor. Good gracious! Don't go doing something from these pages and fuddle a flange or something, then blame us.

Carole, Sam, and Jim persuaded me to try the liver-flush and coffee-enema cleansing and an account of my experience with it may help give you an idea of what to expect.

At first your nose wrinkles up at the thought of these flushes, but if you are strong, common sense overcomes your irrational reluctance. What's so strange? Didn't Grandma always urge a 'good cleaning out' with apples and Epsom salts every now and then? One of the first things my grandmother used to do when I started showing symptoms of being 'sick' as a kid was to give me an enema. Hated it! But it did seem to help.

My first liver flush, and most of my flushes every two months since that somewhat curious beginning in 1980, brought out — terribly personal, mind you — a couple of dozen or more 'greenies'. These are hard, organic stones that just lie around accumulating in the body. They don't do it any good, you can be sure.

Carole poured what seemed like endless glasses of apple juice for me for five days — actually several per day. She was careful to pick a 'natural' brand with no additives, preservatives, or extra sugar. I'm not crazy about apple juice, but my body tolerates it well. And why not — it's tolerated junk well all these years! At least I thought so.

Then, on the sixth day, using our own stylized version of Kelley's suggested procedure, I opened the morning with three doses of Epsom salt, fifteen or twenty minutes apart. Ghastly stuff! Later, feeling drained and thirsty, albeit because of the relief from a case of edema caused by my coffee drinking, Carole fed me fresh fruits and raw (unpasteurized) whipped cream — surprisingly sweet stuff even without honey or sugar. I could eat all of this concoction I wanted. Kelley has special instructions for special cases, such as hypoglycemics, so again we urge you to research this with your doctor before trying it.

Finally, when bedtime rolled around, Carole sympathetically handed me a half cup of raw, unrefined olive oil to drink. The stuff revolts her, and she takes obvious pains to get it down, but I gulped it down in one swoosh, wiped my lips and grinned. She practically gagged at the sight, but I felt fine. No worse than a pint of raw oysters! Again, there are a myriad ramifications, so Kelley literature and other precautions are necessary.

After downing the olive oil, I had to lie down on my right side with my right knee pulled up to my chest. For me, that's not easy. I stayed in that miserable position for half an hour. Kelley explains that this 'encourages the oil to drain from the stomach, helping contents of the gall-bladder and/or liver to move into the small intestine. It does, believe me! In the morning my habitual coffee enema (yes, I think they are addictive) probably wasn't necessary to help me eliminate the hard green stones.

I've often fantasized gathering up the products of my liver flush and having some fun by rushing down to some clinic and complaining that 'these things came out of me! What should I do?' What do you suppose the orthodox physician's reaction would be? Would he immediately offer to operate? Or would he shrug and tell me I'm lucky they didn't get stuck? It's an interesting question to ponder. Kelley, incidentally, reports that his program has never encountered a 'stuck' gallstone. The duct is smallest at the end attached to the gall-bladder, and the relaxed muscles have no difficulty passing the material.

Next, the colon. I've heard it a thousand times if I've heard it once at health conventions: 'Death begins in the colon', many old experts preach. Notice, these experts were invariably 'old', something we all want to live to be, though we won't always admit it.

Today's life-style isn't any easier on our colons than it is on our livers. Our 'sterile' societies kill bacteria with reckless abandon. Food preservatives prevent bacteria from spoiling the merchandize — but the same chemicals may also kill the body's friendly bacteria, which live symbiotically in the lower digestive tract. High-protein diets combined with lack of exercise and other problems already mentioned have 'turned most people's colons into cesspools', says Kelley. The way we live and eat has helped replace the friendly bacteria with putrefying, disease-causing organisms. Most of us walk around every day with low-level ptomaine poisoning in our colons. Add to this factor a lack of fiber in the diet, and our colons are in deep trouble.

Doctors will testify that they don't see any robustly healthy colons in patients over fifty. My own colon, at forty-four, was unspeakable. Diverticuli were diagnosed, and I was on the verge of diverticulosis, which is just about to the point of painful diverticulitis. Carole's fiber-rich natural diet and coffee enemas came to my rescue. Yes, they appear to be habit-forming. They make me feel better.

The problems caused by a malfunctioning ileocecal valve send many a sufferer to the chiropractor (if not to the hospital). The ileocecum is the connective valve between the small intestine and the colon. It lets digested matter pass into the colon while keeping harmful bacteria and other unwanted matter out of the small intestine. One feels terrible when the ileocecal is 'open', allowing a reverse flow of all that waste material and bacteria.

Kelley practitioners instruct people in the art of pressing fingers in the abdomen to close an open ileocecal valve, and most chiropractors show patients how to do it. Many experts in alternative health care recommend high-pressure colonics for cleansing the colon, but Kelley stresses that the enemas are adequate.

Kelley's program concentrates on detoxification for very good reasons. His technicians and the Kelley Book explain in detail the functions of 'purging' the system, fasting to help cleanse, cleaning the kidneys and lungs, and even irrigating the nostrils.

It's impossible to cover everything in Kelley's Metabolic Ecology program, which required twenty years of hard labor to produce, in this book, but we can skim the high points of the remaining aspects of detoxification for you.

Purging refers to the use of Epsom salt, a tablespoon dissolved in two to four ounces of warm distilled water, taken three times, about a half-hour apart, shortly after rising. I combined this purging technique with the liver-gall-bladder flush, but not when I utilized step two of a purge. This is making and drinking an 'alkalizing punch'. To make this punch following Kelley instructions, one mixes the juice of six lemons, six grapefuits, and a dozen oranges with distilled water — one gallon all told. No food or supplements are eaten during a two-day purge. Following the purge, a two-day fast is suggested. However, a Kelley fast is not one of total abstinence. You may have one quart of carrot juice (or grape, cherry, or apple juice if carrot is not available) and all the distilled water you want.

'It is important to remember', Kelley says, 'that unless sufficient fluids are taken, the poisons become concentrated and are not eliminated in the natural way. The coffee enema should be taken once or twice during the day of fasting.'

He adds that potato-peel broth, which is high in potassium, is helpful on a day of fasting and may be taken if desired.

There are other elaborate instructions and suggestions for severe hypoglycemics and for balancing the acid-alkaline situation and for restoring intestinal flora (friendly bacteria).

When it comes to cleansing the kidneys, Kelley is again adamant about the problems generated by our modern life-style:

> The kidneys are vital organs of detoxification. They filter approximately 4,000 quarts of blood daily. The metabolic wastes, largely urea, are eliminated and the acid/alkaline balance maintained. Many drugs are eliminated through the kidneys, especially the common pain-killing drugs which can be extremely damaging to these organs. Such drugs include aspirin, phenacetin and acetominophen. People often don't experience any symptoms from loss of kidney function until 90% of the function is gone, and then the damage is irreversible.

Kelley stresses that America's water supplies are a polluted disgrace, and he won't get much argument from knowledgeable persons. He objects to fluoridated and chlorinated water as stressful to the kidneys and potential health hazards despite what you may have heard to the contrary. He insists upon using pure distilled water (steam-distilled, not merely run through a de-ionizing process) for all cooking, drinking, and enemas. He also recommends certain herb teas (parsley tea is excellent for strengthening the kidneys, he notes) and diuretic foods, such as watermelon on a 'diuretic salad' of garlic, cabbage, and onions. Diuretics are chemical agents that increase the volume of urine. The intake and outflow of water into our bodies is so vitally important to health that the entire next chapter is devoted to drinking water.

Finally, Kelley delves into cleaning the lungs, and he points out that 'the lungs give off many gaseous wastes' as well as carry out the vital oxygen-carbon dioxide cycle. Sometimes a person who starts the Kelley program, or those close to him, may notice a foul odor on his breath. No amount of toothpaste or mouthwash will remove it for long, since it comes from the bloodstream. One can be assured, however, that this is only a phase and that the poisons are leaving the body.

Excess or abnormal mucus is the bane of the breathing apparatus. The detoxifying functions of the lungs are inhibited when mucus clogs the nostrils and/or the bronchial tubes. Kelley says that mucus-forming foods should be avoided if this is a problem. These include 'dairy products, with the exception of butter and cream, and baked flour products, especially white flour. Anti-mucus foods such as raw onions and garlic, cayenne pepper, freshly ground black pepper, fresh ginger and horseradish should be eaten liberally.'

Kelley winds up the detoxification section with brief discussions about irrigating the nostrils, breathing exercises, improving posture, cleaning skin, and acquiring protection against heavy-metal poisoning and radiation. Even in the seemingly innocuous areas there can be controversy. Dr Maynard M. Murray, with whom I co-authored a book on the use of sea salts as fertilizers and as nutrients for hydroponic farming, had been an ear, nose, and throat specialist for decades before leaving his practice for full-time hydroponic farming. Dr Murray told me, in no uncertain terms, that 'sloshing the nostrils with water is one of the worst things anyone can do. Those nose membranes and hairs have natural protections that shouldn't be washed out.' Kelley's research, on the other hand, indicates that cleansing the nostrils can be helpful when done properly. (In fact, yogis and the other practitioners of Ayurveda — the ancient medicine of India — have been doing it for centuries to good effect.)

Breathing exercises from various yoga programs can also be beneficial. And when it comes to posture, I've never found anything better than the Alexander technique, a program developed by Mattias Alexander, an English actor.

Protecting yourself from heavy-metal pollution is simply good sense. Kelley recommends the book *The Poisons around Us*, by Harry Schroeder, M.D. Those who live in urban areas or near heavily traveled highways are exposed to high concentrations of lead. Cigarette smoke, whether your own or someone else's, spews cadmium into the environment. Dentists and their assistants get far more than their share of mercury. (And recent research, such as that by Dr Harold Huggins, shows that mercury leaking from mercury almalgam fillings may cause a wide variety of problems to dental patients.) In modern city living most of us are unknowingly exposed to aluminum, lead, mercury, cadmium, molybdenum, and arsenic. According to Kelley, 'the two factors which have been found most important in helping the body eliminate these poisons are natural food and exercise. Even people who jog in traffic have less lead in their systems than people living in the same area who don't exercise.'

Kelley stresses that certain foods are particularly good for chelation, a process of chemically bonding that draws heavy metals out of the body. 'Dried beans of all kinds are high in the sulphur-containing amino acids which help to remove lead. Garlic, when raw, is high in biologically active selenium and helps to remove cadmium and mercury. Apple pectin and alfalfa sprouts are also helpful.'

In summary, Kelley's years of research clearly indicate that detoxification is every bit as important to your health as nutrition.

Chapter Nine:

Water, Water Everywhere . . .

Early in his research, Kelly insisted that persons undergoing his full detoxificationn program drink and cook with only steam-distilled water, but he had nothing against a good, clean mineral water for general use. Now, however, Kelley contends that steam-distilled or reverse osmosis-filtered water is best for everyone living in today's environment.

Water is immensely interesting stuff, and absolutely vital to life and health, yet we take it for granted in our everyday lives. Chemically, water, associated with life, is inorganic. It is the universal solvent: more substances dissolve in water than in anything else, and many substances that will not dissolve in water, will form a colloidal suspension with it. Substances in solution or colloidal suspension react, chemically, much more rapidly than substances that are not. It is likely that every metabolic reaction in our bodies takes place between substances that are in solution or colloidal suspension. Water, pure water, is vital to our health and well-being. We can survive up to sixty days without food, but only about three days without water.

Note the use of the term *pure water*. The condition of drinking water the world over is increasingly suspect these days, if not downright disgraceful. The alarm has been sounded regarding water pollution, but, curiously, there doesn't appear to be any genuine impetus toward implementing full-scale, practical measures to solve the problem.

Mineral water advocates argue that the body absorbs and uses the trace elements suspended in the water. Most health enthusiasts like to point to the Hunza, an isolated ethnic group in Asia's Caucasus Mountains, who are often cited as the healthiest, longest-lived people on earth. Among other things, the Hunza drink mountain stream water so rich in minerals as to be colored white or slate gray.

Distilled water advocates, however, point out that our bodies have ingested and absorbed so many impurities that we *must* drink only pure water. They say our kidneys are overworked as it is.

The Kelley literature cites Oliver Cabana, Jr., a famed health and nutrition personality from the 1920s and '30s, who wrote: 'There is no calcareous or mineral matter whatsoever in distilled water. Not only do you at once discontinue any possibility of calcareous matter getting into your body through the medium of water you drink, but distilled water has a strong affinity for minerals and it dissolves and carries away a considerable part of the minerals previously in the body.'

The Kelley Book also quotes Dr Edward Elmer Keeler, president of the International Health League:

> The minerals in ordinary drinking water act as irritant poisons to thousands. In distilled water you have a drink that is pure. That is what you need — pure water — not water plus mud, clay, marl, limestone and all manner of animal, vegetable and mineral debris which the kidneys must eliminate. As you begin to use distilled water, you will not only remove all irritation from the kidneys, but increase the purity of the blood and thus aid in rebuilding for health and strength not only the kidneys, but all organs of the body.

These distilled advocates remind us how horrified we might become were we to peer through a powerful microscope at the water spilling forth from our household taps. The number of impurities is immense. Cabana also warned that 'while it takes you only a moment to drink a glass of water, it causes your kidneys to work incessantly, day and night, to strain out these foreign bodies.' Cabana used to preach that 'drugs may stimulate, but distilled water cures.'

Kelley emphasizes that many people forget the ice cubes they make and the water for cooking during their busy daily routines. *All* the water going into your body should be pure, he advises.

The Kelley literature adds that modern deionization processes (cheaper than steam distilling) are 'quite acceptable'. However, if you purchase pure water, be sure glass bottles are used and not plastic. 'Water absorbs harmful chemicals from the plastic and the whole purpose is then defeated.' Sales of home distillation units are increasing steadily in the United States, indicating that many people are taking the message about drinking and cooking water to heart.

After years of testing the results of various water-purification processes, the Kelley Foundation team has finally decided (as of late summer 1985) that the cleanest, least contaminated, most cost-efficient method of getting pure water into a household is through the use of reverse osmosis filtration. The special membrane fibers for the process were invented by DuPont's corporate researchers in the late sixties.

'It is best and least costly to purchase one of the easy-to-install units that fits directly over a tap and requires only about forty pounds of pressure to operate efficiently,' Kelley explained.

The units recommended by the Kelley Foundation feature a five-micron fabric prefilter that removes large particles of rust, scale, dirt, sand and muck from tap water. This prefilter extends the life of the reverse-osmosis membrane, which is capable of filtering out virus, bacteria, other parasites, and chemicals. The reverse-osmosis membrane is followed by a carbon-polishing filter (activated charcoal) and the tap water — regardless of the source — becomes pure and 'tasty'.

No electrical power is required, and the unit lasts for several years. In the United States such units retail for about $300.

Kelley's people prefer the reverse-osmosis system to steam distillation, because the family of chemicals called trihalomethanes that have found their way into many water-supply systems around the world have the same or a lower boiling point than water and are therefore not affected by the distillation process.

Many advocates of mineral water argue that drinking distilled water on a regular basis will deplete the body of vital minerals. Kelley insists that the minerals removed from the body by imbibing pure water are the 'destructive, inorganic minerals that cause, among other things, inflammation of the kidneys, thickened joints, painful nerves, weakened arteries, valvular diseases of the heart, apoplexy, rheumatism and various disturbances of the circulation. Distilled water *never* takes out the organic minerals used by the body for metabolism.'

The preponderance of the evidence seems tilted in favor of pure water, but internationally famous health spas featuring heavily mineralized water for bathing and drinking would certainly disagree.

Perhaps more research into the relative merits of distilled and mineral waters will be undertaken one of these days. It is difficult to abdicate entrenched thinking about mineral water despite the reasonableness of the distilled water arguments. I recall my father telling me that a small amount of sea water ingested every now and then was 'good for me', and it is difficult to ignore a minor fable from Australia concerning ocean water. An elderly couple, he 104 and she 100, were interviewed on one of those standard media events on a hundredth birthday. When asked the secret of their longevity, the couple pointed to the South Indian Ocean just below them and claimed that 'one-quarter cup of sea water every week' was their particular secret.

Well, whatever research into the merits of water may bring, I'd bet that some people would do well on distilled, while others do better on mineral water, depending upon their biochemical individuality.

Despite the uncertainty of the drinking water controversy, we do know for certain that water tainted with microbes — bacteria, viruses, protozoa, fungi, or algae — can make us awfully sick, regardless of our individuality and general state of health. It takes a colony of millions of organisms to seriously infect a healthy body, but if we give them enough of a population base, they'll get us.

Kelley warns that our complacency about the sanitation of public water supplies is simply not warranted. While it's true that science and sanitation engineering have curtailed many of the scourges of yesteryear (typhus, for example), new scourges may be on the horizon. Kelley's literature quotes from U.S. congressman Jim Wright's *The Coming Water Famine:*

Pollution from ordinary sewage and related organic substances is perhaps the worst with which we have to contend. There are fifty-nine million Americans living in approximately two thousand cities who use sewer systems which are either partly or totally inadequate in their treatment of human wastes before those wastes are dumped into rivers and streams. Among these are some of our very largest cities. We have never attacked this, one of the most primitive problems of civilization, with sufficient boldness and forethought.

In addition to human waster, major rivers around the world are contaminated by effluvia from slaughterhouse operations. The Mississippi near St. Louis, Missouri, for example, runs red with blood and entrails from chicken-packing operations along Gravois Creek.

Man seems to have somewhere obtained the inane idea that a flowing stream somehow magically cleans waste. Perhaps animal wastes in purely natural states are readily absorbed and cleansed by the environment, but not tons upon tons of blood and guts. It's certainly no secret that the Missouri features sickening effluent from slaughterhouse activity at Omaha, St. Joseph, and Kansas City, or that the Connecticut River has been perverted into a stinking filth conduit. According to Kelley, one sampling of the Connecticut revealed 'the bacteria of typhoid, paratyphoid, cholera, salmonellosis, tuberculosis, anthrax, tetanus and all the known viruses, including polio, and the tape, round, hook, and pin worms as well as blood flukes.'

Kelley is appalled at the condition of many American waterways. The Kelley Book states: 'With all our vaunted technology, we treat our sewage, on the whole, far less scientifically than do the reputedly backward coolies of the rice paddies of the Orient. After centuries of progress and civilization, we live in greater filth than alley cats in the slums of Calcutta. We still make open latrines of rivers from which others must draw their drinking water.'

Is it any wonder he advocates distilled water?

Don't we kill all those dangerous germs with chlorine? You might ask. Yes, we do — but our war against microbes has created problems of another kind. Trying to create a 'sterile' world has many drawbacks. Dr Bernard Dixon, a British microbiologist who wrote *Invisible Allies: Microbes and Man's Future,* in the mid-1970s, provided a thought-provoking insight into the microscopic world where man literally has more allies than enemies. Modern medical science, of course, didn't see it that way, and we have, over the past 70 years, lived through the decades of 'the microbe hunters', who set out to exterminate the world population of dangerous germs. It's true that science has greatly diminished epidemics of terrible diseases by chemically treating water supplies and by sanitizing much of our sewage, but there must be a better way to 'purify' drinking water than chlorine. Chlorine may be contributing to other serious health problems — problems of a metabolic and chronic nature.

There are a number of better ways to purify water than to use the toxic halogen that makes swimming pools stink with chemical sterility. One excellent method that I encountered as a reporter in Chicago in the mid-1970s was a process called 'photozone.' It utilized ultraviolet light to manufacture 'reactive oxygen' of single oxygen atoms. (Normal oxygen is two atoms of oxygen linked together; single oxygen atoms do not exist except for microseconds in the atmosphere.) This reactive O_1, according to the inventors, bubbled into the water and purified it, and a by-product of pure oxygen emitted from the water's surface. It proved to be economically superior to chlorination, but the chemical lobby in the state of Illinois saw to it that the laws on water 'purification' related especially to chlorine content. Chlorination is everywhere in the modern world.

Joseph M. Price, M.D., in his book *Coronaries, Cholesterol and Chlorine*, presented evidence that the chlorination of water may be a key factor in severe hardening of the arteries (atherosclerosis). He wrote:

Chlorination gained relatively wide acceptance in the 1920s. It was found that satisfactory killing of organisms was dependent upon a residue of chlorine in the water above the amount necessary to react with organic impurities. When it is remembered that evidence of clinical disease from atherosclerosis has taken 10 to 20 years to develop, it becomes evident that there is a correlation between the introduction of widespread application of chlorination of water supplies and the origin and increasing incidence of heart attacks that is exceedingly difficult to explain away.

Apparently there is a direct causal correlation between the amount of chlorine ingested and the speed and degree of development of atherosclerosis, a direct causal relationship that's pretty strong condemnation of a chemical almost everyone else in the country considers perfectly safe.

Chlorine has been shown to destroy vitamin E in the human body. The study was done in 1949 and published in Bridge's *Dietetics for the Clinician.*

Kelley points out that an additional bit of evidence incriminating chlorine in heart disease comes from the writing of W. F. Von Oettingen, M.D., in a book titled *Poisoning.* Oettingen wrote: 'It has been claimed that the injury of the mitral valve of the heart and cardiac insufficiency may result from severe exposure to chlorine, or carbon monoxide. Coronary thrombosis, characterized by palpitation irregularities of the heartbeat and anxiety, has been reported in poisonings with chlorine, carbon monoxide and ferric chloride.'

Kelley also points out that in the case of chlorination of general water supplies the machinery for the process is not as sophisticated as the machinery for adding that other dangerous halogen, fluoride. 'With chlorine,' Kelley stresses, 'there is an unscientific sledgehammer treatment. Large amounts are dumped in at one time.'

And that leads to the other controversial additive in general water systems in much of the modern world — fluoride. Many modern communities throughout the English-speaking world have been convinced that the fluoridation of drinking water protects tooth enamel, thereby helping to prevent dental caries. This is highly controversial in the United States, with the pro-fluoride establishment currently holding the upper hand politically, but not necessarily rationally. Millions of words have been written on the fluoridation controversy, and political battles have raged in numerous American communities over the practice of fluoridating a local city water supply.

It's a huge controversy that we can't delve into here, but we do want to share some rather obscure information with you on the subject. The dawning of the age of fluoride followed shortly after World War II, when the news media boasted about the 'town without a toothache', Hereford, Texas, in the renowned panhandle district. The Texas panhandle plains feature southern dark brown soils, much of it wind-deposited loess. According to a fascinating book on ecologically sound bio-agriculture, the *ACRES USA Primer*, published by Charles Walters, Raytown, Missouri:

> This soil is blessed with a good amount of apatite, which chemically is phosphorus, calcium and fluorine. When apatite decomposes by weathering within the soil, fluorine is the most soluble. It has but a single valence and therefore moves off into the ground water. Calcium has a double valence, or higher combining power, and is therefore less soluble and less active.
>
> Phosphorus has a triple valence, and is the least soluble. As fluorine goes out, calcium and phosphosrus combine to become available to crop plants. It was because of this excellent crop support that the panhandle produced sound teeth and healthy skeletons.
>
> Industries with great overloads of sodium fluoride to get rid of had their scientists conclude that it was the fluorine in the water that made Hereford a town without a toothache — and thus was born the drive to fluoridate the nation's public water supply.

Hereford, it should be noted, is the home of Arrowhead Mills, one of the nation's largest and most successful organic food producers.

The fluoride issue is so heated, and detoxification so vital to health, and pure water so essential to everyone, that we are taking the liberty of repeating some more information from the *ACRES USA Primer*. The writer of this particular excerpt is John R. Lee, M.D.:

> Fluoride is a uniquely potent enzyme poisoner, in fact the most powerful of all the elements. There are several reasons for this. In the table of elements, fluorine belongs to the halogen family, sharing chemical properties with its close relatives, chlorine,

bromine and iodine. As ions reacting with other particles, they all carry one negative charge. As the halogen having the smallest atomic weight, fluoride is naturally the most active. It is extremely active in combining with any element or molecule having a positive valence, such as the mineral ions (enzyme co-factors).

It decomposes water to form hydrogen fluoride which readily attacks glass. It actively replaces its sibling halogen, chlorine, in any solution, including the hydrochloric acid within our stomachs, or any chlorine-containing molecule within our blood or our intracellular fluid. [And, what else is in our public water, abundantly? Chlorine!]

Fluoride's negative charge and atomic weight of 19 is almost identical to the negative charge and weight of the hydroxyl group (OH), 17.008, which is vitally important to the chemical composition of innumerable substances throughout the human organism. It is, in fact, such interchangeability with the hydroxyl group that is cited as the reason for increased hardness of the apatite crystal of tooth enamel when fluoride is involved.

Unfortunately, and all too obviously, this structural change is not confined to the teeth, but occurs elsewhere in the body as well . . . .

And it's not healthful to have fluoride constructions going on elsewhere in our bodies. Teeth need to be hard, but arteries do not; calcium spurs are painfully hard in places they're not meant to be. Both fluoride and chlorine have been cited by various researchers as being contributors to the number-one killer of modern times — atherosclerosis. The big guns from the medical establishment say it isn't so, that evidence does not exist proving that these halogens do dastardly things to soft tissue, but you keep watching the statistics around the world and then mark your ballot for who may be correct.

Before moving on to other aspects of drinking water, we want to share some poignant information regarding fluoridation of public water supplies. This is taken, with permission, from the March 12, 1984 issue of *Spotlight*, a weekly newspaper published in Washington D.C. (see Bibliography). The author of this particular piece was Dr K. A. Baird, a Canadian physician:

Many thought that thalidomide was safe. It wasn't. Before you let your physician be used to support fluoridation of drinking water as safe for everybody, should you not be able to answer the following questions affirmatively?

Have I read one scientific article about the medical aspects of fluoridation?

Do proponents of this mass medication have all the known facts?

Have they done any real research on possible harmful effects?

According to many prominent scientists, biochemists, enzymologists, medical doctors and dentists, the answer to those last two questions is no. They have evidence that fluoridation of public water supplies is wrong.

In 1966 about 200 such persons in London signed a letter, one paragraph of which stated: 'It is our opinion that published research has shown clearly that the toxic effects of fluorides, even in trace quantities, are such that fluoridated drinking water may be harmful, even dangerous, to many people, particularly in its long-term effects, which have not been sufficiently investigated, and that it is therefore quite wrong to force everyone to consume artificially fluoridated water.'

They suggested that children may be given measured individual doses, by medical prescription only.

Hundreds of scientific reports show fluoride as a selective and cumulative poison. Notes on only a few follow:

Eight drug companies warn that their tablets, containing only one milligram of fluoride, can cause skin, stomach, bowel and nervous disorders, headache, vomiting, eczema, atopic dermatitis, urticaria and delayed eruption of teeth . . .

Nobel Prize winner Dr Theorell alone persuaded the Swedish imperial Diet to make fluoridation illegal by telling what he knew about its damage to enzymes . . .

A time lapse film is available showing damage to animal cells caused by one part fluorine in 20 million.

Use of fluoridated Ottawa city water in artificial kidney machines was accompanied by certain bone diseases, spontaneous fractures, weak muscles, nerve irritation, and a vague metabolic disorder . . .

Improvement was prompt when fluoride-free water was used. Simliar observations by Taves . . . illustrated the cumulative tendency of fluoride . . . .

We've excerpted portions of the lengthy article to make a point, and we assume it is made. However, to add just one more brand to the fire, the accompanying table, taken from the same issue of *Spotlight*, may tell something about the view of fluoridation in the non-English-speaking world.

Countries Reject Poison

You are constantly bombarded with pro-fluoridation propaganda. But if fluoride is so good, wouldn't it be used around the world? Following is a list of some countries where fluoridation has been suggested and the results.

Country and Population	Status of Fluoride	Action or Comment
Austria 7,500,000	No fluoridation	Will not be carried out.
Belgium 9,750,000	No fluoridation	Only one small experimental plant, now discontinued.
Denmark 5,000,000	No fluoridation	Forbidden by law in food and water.
Egypt 37,230,000	No fluoridation	U.S. pressure to fluoridate. Rejected.
France 52,000,000	No fluoridation	Never considered essential to good health.

Country and Population	Status of Fluoride	Action or Comment
Germany 61,000,000	No fluoridation	Discontinued in 1971 after 18 years of experiments 'for health and legal reasons.'
Greece 9,000,000	No fluoridation	No experimental programs have ever been introduced.
Holland 13,500,000	No fluoridation	Discontinued in 1976 after 23 years of experiments involving 9 million citizens. On August 31, 1976, by royal decree, all permissions to fluoride were canceled.
India 598,170,000	No fluoridation	Endemic fluorosis occurs with varying intensity in many parts of India. The removal of fluoride from water is a major public health problem. Defluoridation units are functioning in parts of India.
Italy 55,000,000	No fluoridation	In some areas public drinking water supplies are defluoridated.

Country and Population	Status of Fluoride	Action or Comment
Luxembourg 360,000	No fluoridation	
Norway 4,000,000	No fluoridation	Legislation designed to make fluoridation compulsory was rejected by the Norwegian Parliament in 1975.
Spain 35,000,000	No fluoridation	Forbidden by law.
Sweden 8,200,000	No fluoridation	Forbidden by law. Discontinued in 1969 after a 10-year experimental program. The World Health Organization was asked to produce evidence to support its earlier claim that fluoridation was 'safe'. No evidence was produced. Parliament declared fluoridation illegal on November 18, 1971.
Switzerland 6,500,000	One experimental program only since 1959, and it serves just four percent of the total population. In December, 1975, the Swiss Health Department advised the cessation of fluoridation in Switzerland 'due to its ineffectiveness'.	

Reprinted from *Spotlight*, March 12, 1984, with permission.

In the Kelley Book, this is what you'll learn about fluoridated water:

As for fluorine treatment, research indicates, beyond a shadow of a doubt, that fluoridation of water and foods, and other ingestion of fluorides into the body, is extremely harmful and often fatal. Homeopathic physicians have found that fluoride in doses of one part per million (the amount commonly used in fluoridation) is a harmful dose of medication and that continued use acts as a violent poison, with serious physical and psychological effects. Fluoride is one of the major causes of obesity, interfering with the function of the thyroid gland and all the enzyme systems of the body. This is one of the reasons why diet drinks, which generally contain fluoride, aren't as helpful in reducing weight as people would like them to be. Fluoride is also a contributing cause of abnormally tall growth among young people and of abnormally broad bottoms among women. All bodily processes are adversely affected by the use of fluoride. There is no unprejudiced evidence that fluoride is helpful in cavity prevention. Scientific evidence is that magnesium in the water, not fluoride, is what reduces cavities.

Finally, as though we haven't frightened you enough, there is one other key water-poisoning activity foisted onto nature by arrogant Man, and this one may be the worst of all in the long run. The greatest single source of water pollution on earth — worldwide — is run off from precipitation (rain, snow) that carries with it silt and all the petrochemicals used by modern agriculture. Streams, rivers, lakes, and even the oceans are beginning to crawl with the residue from herbicides and pesticides sprayed liberally every year over farmlands all over the world. Synthetic-organic chemicals, such as pesticides, herbicides, chemical fertilizers, synthetic rubbers, detergents, dyes, and the like are virtually insoluble in water and are impervious to most present-day techniques in water purification.

Consider this: The single greatest agricultural problem, worldwide, is the loss of topsoils to erosion. Now, what has been washed away with those topsoils year in and year out? Poisons, like DDT, banned (allegedly) by the United States and other enlightened nations, are still used indiscriminately in many parts of the world. An incident several decades ago, in which sea birds were severely damaged by DDT residue reaching their habitat, should have taught the world a lesson not easily forgotten. Evidently, humanity has a short memory.

Wise people will spend the extra money to purchase bottled distilled water or to install home purification equipment. It is best, and more cost-efficient, to buy a unit and purify from your own tap. Kelley warns: 'If distilling from a city water supply, remember that certain hydrocarbon contaminants have a lower boiling point than that of water. The distilling unit should have a valve to permit their escape as they gasify. If not, they will concentrate in the distilled water and will need to be removed by filtering through activated charcoal.'

Finally, let's look at what has been called 'Willard Water', in the United States, thanks to the popularity of the television show *60 Minutes*, which featured the story of Dr John W. Willard, Sr., and his claims for his patented 'catalyst altered water'. Today anyone can buy small amounts of 'CAW' from Dr Willard's company in Rapid City, South Dakota, or from other companies (some of which are being sued for alleged infringements by Willard).

To tell you precisely what catalyst activated water is will take some doing. It's a relatively easy concept for chemists, but we uninitiated lay persons may have some trouble. It's simple, but it's not easy. Willard Water is 'wetter water', but not in the same sense as 'softer' water or the slick-feeling water we feel when we plunge our dishpan hands into a basin of suds, which is also, in a sense, wetter water.

Water is the universal solvent, and Dr Willard's chemical discovery, he says, catalyzes ordinary distilled water into, for want of a better term, 'supersolvent'. Now, water molecules are tiny crystals, and they tend to clump and agglute and stick together making water 'hard'. Our detergent manufacturers know that soap or detergent cleans grime better (the solvent quality of water is enhanced) when water is 'softer', so they break up the hardness of water with chemical 'surfactants'. A surfactant simply breaks the surface tension of water. (You can observe the surface tension of water in the beads of water droplets on your automobile's waxy surface before you wipe them away.)

Willard feels that his water has more than mere surfactant acitivity; it has a catalytic activity that gives water molecules more pizazz, making the water more readily useful to your body. The scientific world has balked at these claims, and the evidence at this time is empirical — if the wonder water works, nobody knows why; if it fails, nobody knows why!

Carole and our sons are convinced that Willard Water gives them 'more energy', and after about a year's use they miss it if it's not available. As usual my body doesn't give me a clue whether Willard's Water is doing me any good, but when it comes to burns on our skin, our entire family has empirical evidence that the catalyst activated water does something good. Carole has found that by spraying Willard Water over a chemical burn with a misting device she knocked out the pain and eliminated the redded area within a day. Sunburn is soothed by Willard Water mist, and when I spilled boiling water on my wrist, I used the Willard Water spray and enjoyed the experience. It hurt as burns always hurt, so I sprayed and the pain went away — but ice may have done the same, or any cool water, you say. Not so! I used ice, and the moment I raised the ice from the welt, the pain was back; with Willard spray the pain stayed away after the spray for a long period, perhaps ten- to fifteen-minute periods for the first two hours, then for longer periods through the night, No dressing, no nothing other than the CAW mist, and the next day no welts, no blisters! Not even aloe vera, my old burn standby, ever worked so well.

Why? I can only guess. The catalyst activated water was taken readily into the burned area and did a job that ordinary water could not do. Incidentally, I've long been an advocate of water for burns, even when people were still smearing butter or petroleum jelly on them.

Before presenting Willard's reasoning about his own invention, here's a little background from my journalistic bag of tricks that has never before been in print. About ten years ago, I met one of the world's most inventive minds, and he became one of my best friends. G. G. Gatling of North Carolina (his great granduncle Richard Gatling invented the machine gun) is as unsophisticated and as 'backwoodsy' as a rural American can get. His insights and inventive genius bring him into contact with all kinds of unusual people and things. One of the encounters he shared with me, was 'Mac's water'. Mac — Russell McDaniel of Felt, Oklahoma — boasted about and sold a product for growing crops called Mac-T-Vator, and like another Willard product, XXX water, it is primarily for plants. The special water is good for plant growth, health, and yield, as well as for drought and disease resistance. Mac also claimed his water could do marvelous things for sick people, and to this day G.G. always has some on hand around his home for health purposes. I've heard tales of miracle cures for everything from stomach flu to acne, and even some cancer talk. Unsubstantiated tales they remain, but while I always suspect exaggeration, I've also learned that where there is smoke, there's fire.

The purpose of this digression is to put Willard's heralded innovation into perspective. Willard is evidently not the first to claim to have found a way to enhance the wonder of ordinary water; he's simply the most noted.

Willard's discovery came in stages and began in the 1930s when he sought a better formula for cleaning grease and grime, oil, and hardened carbon off railroad equipment. He learned a lot about water as a solvent during those years as a railroad chemist. Then in 1946 he moved to Rapid City, where he became a chemistry teacher, and through serendipity, and thanks to the abundance of lignite (low-grade coal) in the Dakotas, he evolved his patented catalyst. Willard's literature states: 'It is not known how nor why the nutrients, trace minerals, humic acids and amino acids extracted from lignite by Dr Willard's water are so extremely effective on the growth of plants.'

Because of the U.S. Food and Drug Administration edicts against making health claims, Dr Willard's literature refers to the health benefits that plants receive from the catalyst activated products he makes, and then it stressses that reputable laboratories have analyzed and tested his activated water and found no harmful effects on humans whatsoever.

Carole and I conclude that it can't hurt, and it may help. We don't cook with Willard Water, but we drink it regularly. Who knows, it may be just what the doctor didn't order that solves a problem for your particular metabolic type.

Chapter Ten:

The Future of Metabolic Typing

We have all heard disclaimers that read, 'This program is not for everyone, but . . .' Well, the metabolic typing program *is* for everyone, because it deals with each individual's uniqueness. This does not mean, however, that Kelley's program is without the usual share of controversy. The medical establishment simply does not recognize metabolic typing, but there are numerous signs that changes are on the horizon. No innovation in medical science ever breezed its way into full and prominent acceptance without meeting resistance from the powers that be.

A few critics have voiced opinions that Kelley's program is froth with 'overkill'. They suggest that he prescribes far too many supplements and that his questionnaire is unnecessarily long. We considered these opinions and decided they're not valid based upon our experiences and our investigation. First, Kelley's supplements are not merely large doses of vitamins and minerals. Instead, they are a carefully worked out series of combinations of enzymes, glandulars, and organ derivatives blended with appropriate vitamins and minerals. Second, the supplements are required in adequate amounts for each metabolic type to make up for the surprisingly pronounced shortages in our food. There isn't enough truly organic produce to go around, and today's farmland is depleted of nature's bounty. Most farmland is overchemicalized in an effort to grow more bushels of product. Unfortunately, much of those vast yields are nutritionally inferior as compared with yields of less chemical times. The same essential nourishment missing from farm crops appears to be also missing in the farm animals feeding upon it. Factory farming — the mass production of cattle, pigs, and chickens in unnatural environments — leaves a lot to be desired.

Animals are injected with antibiotics and steroids to enhance profitability without regard to potential health hazards. The hormone DES, formerly injected in beef cattle to improve growth rate, has been outlawed in the United States, but many feedlots have ignored the ban or have simply changed labels on the hormone injections. The animals themselves are so unhealthy they require staggering doses of antibiotics just to make it to market.

In the spring of 1984, I had occasion to interview the late Ralph Engelken of Greeley, Iowa. Engelken's 500-acre farm is one of the largest and most successful 'organic' farms in America. He prefers the term 'bio-agriculture' to 'organic' because the latter refers more to gardening. The Engelken story was interesting, not only because of his twenty-five-year success with natural farming, but also because of the economic trend that may be in the making. Engelken had difficulty with refinancing his farm despite its favorable cash flow. The reason, it was learned, hinged upon the fact that his land, having already eliminated the chemical poisoning conditions, loomed greater in value than the adjacent farmlands where chemicals continued to pollute. Yes, the chemicalized farms — using petrochemical fertilizers instead of manure and humus and pesticides and herbicides galore, are still producing high yields, but . . .

'Corn is not sold by protein content,' Engelken remarked, 'but changes are coming.' Most of Engelken's corn was fed to his livestock in a remarkably successful growth and fattening program. The protein content in Engelken's corn ranges from 9 per cent to 12 per cent. The protein content in all the chemically grown corn ranges from 2 per cent to 5 per cent.

Dr Maynard Murray, the hydroponic sea salt expert I mentioned in a previous chapter, told me that in 1930 an ear of corn would have as many as thirty trace elements present, but today's corn features less than twelve total elements.

Carole, Sam and Jim experimented with the number of supplements their particular programs called for. When they cut back on the suggested amounts, they lost decided advantages in energy and sense of well-being.

Today's denatured, refined, processed, and chemicalized foods, coming from depleted, chemicalized soils, apparently dictate increased supplementation. Yes, it's costly, but the price for health is deemed worth it.

What about the multitude of questions on the questionnaire? Well, it does require patience and fortitude to wade through page after page of multiple-choice questions. But when a person's health is at stake, or a chronic malady threatens, the time and effort needed to get all the information into the computer in order to provide the most reliable, failsafe, metabolic typing data possible are most certainly worth it. The repetition in the questionnaire is there for a reason. Researchers and pollsters have discovered that Americans are not always entirely truthful about what they eat. In order to filter fact from fiction, the Kelley questionnaire is overly comprehensive, thereby catching us when we try to kid ourselves. The repetition also helps to pinpoint particulars rather than settle for vague generalizations about the respondent's individuality.

Kelley, however, is a realist, and he has responded, reluctantly, to the demand for a shorter form. A second metabolic classification program has been worked up to be used by the 'healthy' person who wants merely to supplement his diet while on an exercise program, or merely while attempting to improve his condition. In the short-form metabolic typing program you may determine whether your metabolism lies within one of the three major classifications — sympathetic, parasympathetic, or balanced. The Kelley Institute has fashioned a short form with only a few hundred questions, and from this shortened version the computer will determine which of the three broad classifications matches your metabolism. Once that is established, and the computer data are mailed out to the subscriber, he or she may obtain the supplements designed for the proper classification. I took the short form and learned that my general classification is 'parasympathetic-dominant'. I may now send for my 'P' pack of special nutritional supplements.

Kelley was reluctant to provide the shortened form because people tend to want to use it for seriously diseased conditions, and it would be a mistake to do so. The shorter form simply cannot provide enough detailed information for the computer program to evaluate a diseased condition adequately. For example, on the short form a question reads 'I like fruits,' then offers three choices: 'A lot';

'occasionally'; 'very little'. Now, I don't like fruit, generally speaking, but I consume bananas like the proverbial ape. So how do I respond to the question and give the computer a true picture? As you see, I cannot. The longer questionnaire, with its special categories for men and women separately and its more comprehensively designed questions, can ask fruit by fruit, vegetable by vegetable, bad habit by bad habit, and so forth, thus giving a more detailed picture of the individual metabolism. In instances where chronic disease is concerned, the short form simply will not do, nor will the special supplement packets designed for the generalized short form participants.

As of this writing, the cost of a computerized short form to accompany a physical fitness program, for example, is $50 in the United States. For your money, you will receive a surprisingly comprehensive printout on your general classification. The full Kelley program replete with a trained metabolic therapist, often a physician, ranges between $300 and $400 in the United States. The costs listed here do not include the cost of the supplements, which are expensive since they must attain the high quality demanded by Kelley. The address for the International Health Institute is given at the end of the book.

This book has introduced you to one of the newer and more promising realms of preventive medical theory and practice. Having studied the Kelley program diligently Carole and I conclude that this remarkable researcher has, indeed, found 'medicine's missing link'. Carole and her son Jim have decided to attend Kelley training programs to qualify as metabolic therapists.

Not only does the metabolic typing approach to health make good sense, but Kelley's research appears to have opened the door to a new and exciting way of studying human behaviour. The metabolic type studies have revealed a physiology-of-behavior overview not previously considered by the various schools of psychology.

Kelley and his associates, John W. Rhinehart, M.D. (a psychiatrist), and William L. Wolcott, have begun an intensive research into behavior as it relates to the sympathetic-dominant and parasympathetic-dominant metabolisms. They have observed distinct correlations between type dominance and behavior in the areas of business, education, marriage and family, and general psychology.

For example, in business, research shows that the sympathetic-dominant individual is the 'driving force, logical thinking, action-oriented' executive, while the parasympathetic-dominant is the 'people person' — the manager who gets along with everyone and has an 'intuitive knack' for making decisions.

Once you establish your metabolic type, and perhaps the types of your family, many previously puzzling behavioral patterns may be readily perceived from a physiological rather than a psychological point of view. In our family we were able to understand each other better once we realized that Sam exhibited definite 'sympathetic dominance,' while Jim and I exhibited 'parasympathetic natures'. Carole is balanced, but leaning to sympathetic.

In business, metabolic typing may be tailored to place the right person in the right position. When a parasympathetic-dominant sales manager meets a parasympathetic-dominant purchasor, the sale is virtually assured. However, a sympathetic-dominant executive may find that parasympathetic-dominant tactics drive him up a wall, and vice versa. Balance, of course, also plays a key role, but dominance meeting dominance in the various areas of everyday living provides many of life's so-called psychological problems.

In the classroom, your parasympathetic-dominant child may encounter a sympathetic-dominant teacher, or vice versa. Sympathetic-dominant teachers will tend to be bright, quick, intellectually oriented, and practical. The parasympathetic-dominant child will appear to be a daydreamer, or the chatty child who fails to pay attention. Instant conflict! Something generally called a 'personality conflict' may be described by both parties. However, once a physiological basis can be established behind behavior patterns, solutions to the 'personality conflicts' may become readily available.

Wolcott, Kelley's chief assistant, has found that if you wish to teach a sympathetic-dominant individual something new, you do well to deal with logic and left-brain activity. If you wish to teach a parasympathetic-dominant individual something new, deal with intuition and feeling and right-brain activity.

Marriage poses interesting conflicts, and Wolcott stressed that knowing a prospective mate's metabolic dominance can lead to much smoother sailing and greater understanding. A sympathetic-dominant husband with a parasympathetic-dominant wife fits the traditional marriage ideas of domineering husband and submissive wife. The variables are legion, of course, and the subject promises to expand a thousandfold in the next few years. Meanwhile, just knowing where you stand in the dominance category may help a great deal in better understanding the various 'personality conflicts' that arise in your life.

Now, before you decide that investigating the metabolic typing program is all right for someone else, but you don't need to bother, let's reread the list of statistics and facts you read in Chapter 2:

- 999 out of 1,000 people today are malnourished.
- Birth defects in the U.S. have tripled since 1956.
- About 80 per cent of the modern western world's population suffers from degenerative conditions.
- The National Cancer Institute found that diet and nutrition appear to account for the largest number of human cancers.
- Only a few years ago, accidents were the major cause of death in children under the age of fifteen, but today the number one cause is cancer.
- One person dies of cancer every eighty seconds in the United States.
- Degenerative disease conditions, such as cancer, diabetes, heart disease, hypoglycemia, eczema, emphysema, arthritis, and ulcers occur in more and more *children* each year.
- Chronic illness is responsible for more than 80 percent of the total cases of disability in the U.S. and England.
- Each year the United States drops lower and lower on the list of 'health of nations'.

For further information regarding metabolic typing programs write to:

International Health Institute
P.O. Box 802607
Dallas, Texas 75380

Toll-free telephone in continental
U.S.A.: 1-800-527-0453

To contact Tom and Carole Valentine, write to:

P.O. Box 639
Del Mar, California 92014

MDs in England who administer the Kelley program:

Dorothy West, M.D.
Rutt House
Ivybridge
Devon, England PL21 0DQ

Milo Siewert, M.D.
26 Sea Road
Boscombe, Bournemouth
Dorset, England

Bibliography

The following publications are cited in the Kelley Book as being useful in assembling information contributing to the program. Studying them will help you broaden the understanding of metabolic typing and will serve as additional sources of useful information.

Airola, Paavo O. *Are you Confused?* Phoenix, Ariz.: Health Plus Publishers.

———, *There is a Cure for Arthritis* Phoenix, Ariz.: Health Plus Publishers.

Answer — Preventive Medicine. Anaheim, Calif.: Alsleben Foundation.

Bailey, Herbert. *The Vitamin Pioneers.* New York: Pyramid Publishers.

Bardwell, Lorena. *Modern Meatless Menus.* Baton Rouge, L.: Claitor's Book Store.

Biology of the Trace Elements — Their Role in Nutrition. Philadelphia: J. B. Lippincott.

Blumenfeld, Arthur. *Heart Attack! Are You a Candidate?* New York: Pyramid Publications.

Bowes and Church. *Food Values of Portions Commonly Used.* Philadelphia: J. B. Lippincott.

Bradley, Alice V. *Tables of Food Values.* Peoria, Illi.: Chas. A. Bennett Co.

Bragg, Paul C. *The Shocking Truth about Water.* Burbank, Calif.: Health Science.

Cheraskin, E., and Ringsdorf, W. M. *New Hope for Incurable Diseases.* Jericho, N. Y.: Exposition Press.

Clark, Linda. *Be Slim and Healthy.* New Canaan, Conn.: Keats Publishing.

————, *Light on Your Health Problems.* New Canaan, Conn.: Keats Publishing.

————, *Secrets of Health and Beauty.* New York: Pyramid Publishers.

————, *Stay Young Longer.* New York: Pyramid Publishers.

Composition of Foods. U.S. Dept. of Agriculture, Research Service Handbook No. 8. Washington, D. C.: Government Printing Office.

Council on Foods and Nutrition of the American Medical Association. *Handbook of Nutrition.* Philadelphia: Blakeston Co.

Cox, W. R. *Test Animals — Chinchillas.* Milwaukee, Wis.: Lee Foundation for Nutritional Research.

Crum, Gertrude B. *A World of Menus and Recipes,* Indianapolis and New York: Bobbs-Merrill Co.

Cureton, Thomas K. *The Physiological Effects of Wheat Germ Oil on Humans in Exercise.* Springfield Ill.: Charles C. Thomas, Publisher.

Damerow, Ronald D. *The Right to Live.* New York: Vantage Press.

Daro, A.F.; Gollin, H. A.; and Zivkovic. *Vitamins and Minerals in Obstetrics and Gynecology. International Surgery,* September 1971.

Davidson, Sir Stanley, and Passmore, R. *Human Nutrition and Dietetics.* Baltimore, M.: Williams and Wilkins Co.

Di Cyran, Erwin. *Vitamin E and Aging.* New York: Pyramid Publishers.

Dietary Goals for the United States. United States Senate, Select Committee of Nutrition and Human Needs, 2nd ed., December 1977. Washington, D. C.: Government Printing Office.

Diets Meeting Allowances for Nutrients. U.S. Dept. of Agriculture, Agricultural Research Service, 5907-69 (8). Washington, D. C.: Government Printing Office.

Dintenfass, Julius. *Chiropractic — A Modern Way to Health.* New York: Pyramid Publishers.

Dolger, Henry. *How to Live with Diabetes.* New York: Pyramid Publishers.

Ehret, Arnold. *Mucusless Diet Healing System.* Beaumont, Calif.: Ehret Literature Publishing.

El Molino Best Recipes. Alhambra, Calif.: El Molino Mills.

Facts about Nutrition. U.S. Dept. of Health, Education and Welfare, 1973. Washington, D. C.: Government Printing Office.

Family Fare. U.S. Dept. of Agriculture, Home and Garden Bulletin No. 1, 1971. Washington, D. C.: Government Printing Office.

Fathman, George and Doris. *Live Foods.* Show Low, Ariz.: Sun Haven Enterprises.

Final Report. White House Conference on Food, Nutrition and Health, 1969. Washington, D. C.: Government Printing Office.

Flatto, Edwin. *The Restoration of Health — Nature's Way.* New York: Pyramid Publishers.

Food Facts from Rutgers. New Brunswick, N. J.: Rutgers.

Food Guide for Older Folks. U.S. Dept of Agriculture, Home and Garden Bulletin No. 17. Washington, D. C.: Government Printing Office.

Food Is More Than Just Something to Eat. U.S. Depts. of Agriculture and Health, Education and Welfare, 1975. Washington, D. C.: Government Printing Office.

Food — The Yearbook of Agriculture 1959. Washington, D. C.: Government Printing Office.

Ford, Roberts. *Stale Food vs. Fresh Food.* Pascagoula, Miss.: Magnolia Laboratory.

Guthrie, Helen A. *Introductory Nutrition.* St. Louis, Mo.: C. V. Mosby Co.

Harrower, Henry R. *Practical Endocrinology.* Milwaukee, Wis.: Lee Foundation for Nutritional Research.

Hovannessian, A. T. *Raw Eating.* Tehran: A. R. Hovannessian.

Human Nutrition. Science and Education Staff Report No. 1 and Report No. 2. Washington, D. C.: Government Printing Office.

Human Nutrition, Benefits from Human Nutrition Research, U.S. Dept. of Agriculture, Report No. 2, 1971. Washington, D. C.: Government Printing Office.

Hunter, Beatrice Trum. *Fact Book on Yogurt and Kefir.* New Canaan, Conn.: Keats Publishing.

————, *Food Additives and Your Health.* New Canaan, Conn.: Keats Publishing.

————, *The Natural Foods Cookbook.* New York: Pyramid Publishers.

_____, *The Natural Foods Primer*. New York: Simon & Schuster.

Improving Teenage Nutrition. U.S. Dept. of Agriculture, Federal Extension Service, PA 599. Washington, D. C.: Government Printing Office.

Kervran, Louis C. *Biological Transmutations*. Binghamton, N. Y.: Swan House Publishing Co.

Key Nutrients. U.S. Dept. of Agriculture, Extension Service, PA 691, 1971. Washington, D. C.: Government Printing Office.

Kirschner, H. E., and White, H. C. *Are You What You Ear?* La Sierra, Calif.: H. C. White Publications.

Klenner, Fred R., and Bartz, Fred H. *The Key to Good Health — Vitamin C.* Chicago: Graphic Arts Research Foundation.

Kloss, Jethro. *Back to Eden.* New York: Beneficial Books.

Larson, Gena. *Better Food for Better Babies.* New Canaan, Conn.: Keats Publishing.

_____, *Fundamentals in Foods*. Solana Beach, Calif.: I.A.C.V.F.

Lappé, Frances M. *Diet for a Small Planet.* New York: Ballantine Books.

Let's Live magazine. Los Angeles, Calif.

Light, Louise. *In Praise of Vegetables.* New York: Scribner and Sons.

Lindlahr, Victor H. *You Are What You Eat.* Hollywood, Calif.: Newcastle Publishing Co.

Long, Cyril. *Biochemists' Handbook.* New York: Van Nostrand Reinhold Co.

Longgood, William. *The Poisons in Your Food.* New York: Pyramid Publications.

Loomis, Mildred. *Go Ahead and Live.* New Canaan, Conn.: Keats Publishing.

Lucas, Richard. *Nature's Medicines.* New York: Award Books.

Machek, Otakar. 'The Challenge of Muscular Dystrophy.' La Habra, Calif.: *Journal of Applied Nutrition*, vol. 15.

Magnesium in Human Nutrition, U.S. Dept. of Agriculture, Home Economics Research Report No. 19. Washington, D. C.: Government Printing Office.

Master Herbology. Phoenix, Arix.: Nature's Way Products.

Mayo Clinic Diet Manual. Philadelphia: W. B. Saunders Co.

National Academy of Science — Nutritional Research Council. *Recommended Dietary Allowances,* Revised 1968. Washington, D. C.: N.A.S.

Nearing, Helen and Scott. *Living the Good Life.* New York: Schocken Books.

Norris, P. E. *Everything You Want to Know about Wheat Germ.* Moonachie, N. J.: Pyramid Publications.

————, *Everything You Want to Know about Slimming.* Moonachie, N. J.: Pyramid Publications.

Nichols, Joe D., and Presley, James. *Please Doctor, Do Something!* Atlanta, Tex.: Natural Food Associates.

Nittler, Alan H. *A New Breed of Doctor.* New York: Pyramid House.

Nutrition and Healthy Growth. U.S. Dept. of Health, Education, and Welfare, Welfare Administration, Children's Bureau, Publication 352. Washington, D. C.: Government Printing Office.

Nutrition — Background and Issues. 1971 White House Conference on Aging. Washington, D. C.: Government Printing Office.

Nutrition — Food at Work for You. U.S. Dept. of Agriculture, 1971. Washington, D. C.: Government Printing Office.

Nutrition — Recommended for Action. 1971 White House Conference on Aging. Washington, D. C.: Government Printing Office.

Nutrition Survey, 1968-1970. U.S. Dept. of Health, Education and Welfare Publications 72-8130 through 72-8134. Washington, D.C.: Government Printing Office.

Nutrition — Up to Date Up to You. U.S. Dept. of Agriculture, Human Nutrition Research Division, Agricultural Research Services. Washington, D. C.: Government Printing Office.

Nutritional Status — Select Committee on Nutrition and Human Needs. U.S. Senate, 1974. Washington, D.C.: Government Printing Office.

Nutritive Value of Foods. U.S. Dept. of Agriculture, 1971. Washington, D. C.: Government Printing Office.

Nusz, Frieda. *Natural Foods Blender Cookbook.* New Canaan, Conn.: Keats Publishing.

Orten, James M. and Neuhaus, O. W. *Biochemistry.* St. Louis, Mo.: C. V. Mosby Co.

Page, Melvin E., D.D.S., and Abrams, H. Leon Jr. *Your Body Is Your Best Doctor.* New Canaan, Conn.: Keats Publishing.

Planning for the Later Years. U.S. Dept. of Health, Education, and Welfare, Social Security Administration. Washington, D. C.: Government Printing Office.

Prevention: The Magazine for Better Health. Emmaus, Pa.: Rodale Books.

Price, Joseph M. *Coronaries, Cholesterol and Chlorine.* New York: Pyramid Publishers.

Pugh, Katherine, *Mental Illness: Is It Necessary?* New York: Carlton Press.

Richomond, Sonya. *International Vegetarian Cookery.* New York: Arco Publishing.

Roberts, Sam. E. *Exhaustion — Causes and Treatment.* Emmaus, Pa.: Rodale Books.

Robinson, Corinne H., *Fundamentals of Normal Nutrition.* New York: Macmillan Co.

Rodale J. I. *Natural Health, Sugar and the Criminal Mind.* New York: Pyramid Publications.

———, *Magnesium: The Nutrient That Could Change Your Life.* New York: Pyramid Publications.

———, *Rodale's System for Mental Power and Natural Health.* New York: Pyramid Publications.

Schubert, Brund H. *Survival of Mankind.* Huntington Park, Calif.: Free-Economy Association.

Schultz, Dodi. *Have Your Baby . . . and Your Figure Too.* New York: Pyramid Publishers.

Shelton, Herbert M. *Food Combining Made Easy.* Bonita Springs, Fl.: Shangri-La Health Resort.

Sherman H. E. *Chemistry of Food and Nutrition.* New York: Macmillan Co.

Thomas, Virginia Castleton. *My Secrets of Natural Beauty.* New Canaan, Conn.: Keats Publishing.

Tilden, J. H. *Toxemia Explained.* Mokelumne Hill, Calif.: Health Research.

Tobe, John H. *Romance in the Garden.* Toronto: George J. McLeod, Ltd.

———, *Sprouts — Elixir of Life.* St. Catharines, Canada: Provoker Press.

Toward the New. U.S. Dept. of Agriculture Bulletin 341, 1972. Washington, D. C.: Government Printing Office.

Trace Elements in Human Nutrition. Technical Report Series No. 532, 1973. Geneva: World Health Organization.

Turner, Dorothea. *Handbook of Diet Therapy.* Chicago: University of Chicago Press.

Turner, James S. *Ralph Nader's The Chemical Feast.* New York: Grossman Publishers.

Wade, Carlson. *Fact Book on Vitamins and Other Food Supplements.* New Canaan, Conn.: Keats Publishing.

————, *The Natural Laws of Healthful Living.* New York: Pyramid Publications.

Walker, N. W. *Raw Vegetable Juice.* New York: Pyramid Publications.

————, *Vibrant Health — The Possible Dream.* Phoenix, Ariz.: Norwalk Press.

Warmbrand, Max. *Eat Well to Keep Well.* New York: Pyramid Publishers.

————, *Add Years to Your Heart.* New York: Pyramid Publishers.

Watts, B. K., and Merrill, A.L. *Composition of Foods — Raw, Processed, Prepared,* U.S. Dept. of Agriculture, Bulletin 8. Washington, D. C.: Government Printing Office.

————, *Energy Value of Foods.* U.S. Department of Agriculture, Handbook 74. Washington, D. C.: Government Printing Office.

White, Ellen G. *Counsels on Diet and Foods.* Takoma Park, Washington, D. C.: Review and Herald Publishing Association.

Wohl, Michael C., and Goodhart, R. S. *Modern Nutrition in Health and Disease.* Philadelphia: Lea and Febiger.

The Womanly Art of Breast Feeding. Franklin Park, Ill.: La Leche League International.

Worth, Miklos. *Yoghurt Spells Health.* New York: Ideal Health Books.

Williams, Roger J. *You Are Extraordinary.* New York: Pyramid Publishers.

————, *Alcoholism: The Nutritional Approach.* Austin, Tex.: University of Texas Press.

————, *Nutrition against Disease.* New York: Pitman Publishing.

————, *Nutrition in a Nutshell.* Garden City, N. Y.: Doubleday and Co.